Sir Herbert Duthie Library
Llyfrgell Syr Herbert Duthie

University Hospital
of Wales
Heath Park
Cardiff
CF14 4XN

Ysbyty Athrofaol Cymru
Parc y Mynydd Bychan
Caerdydd
CF14 4XN

029 2074 2875
duthieliby@cardiff.ac.uk

IRWIN M. RUBIN and T.W. BODEN

Dying for Compassion

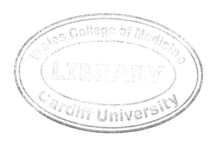

Kingsham Press

First published 2005
by Kingsham Press

Oldbury Complex
Marsh Lane
Easthampnett
Chichester, West Sussex
PO18 0JW
United Kingdom

Typeset in Palatino

Printed and bound by
J. H. Haynes and Co. Ltd.
Sparkford
Nr. Yeovil
Somerset
UK

ISBN: 1-904235-37-9

British Library Cataloguing in Publication Data
A catalogue record of this book is available from the British Library

Rubin, Irwin M. and Boden, T.W.

Dedication

When I sat down to begin this novel, I was vaguely aware of, and accepted as valid, observations others had made in their acknowledgments. The invaluable help of innumerable others and the disclaimers as to their accountability, to name just two, have certainly proven equally true for me. My gratitude to them is detailed in the appropriate section.

What made less sense to me as I began were verbal observations writer friends made to the effect that "Your first novel is likely to be the most autobiographical of any you write (Who could even think beyond the daunting task of one?) and will, therefore, be more gut-wrenching." In blissful ignorance I started on my journey, convinced that their warning was for lesser mortals. No inner voice was going to get the best of me and 'force' me to write anything I didn't want to write. This dedication is proof of that naivete.

I wish I could say that Louis Rubin, my father, was a source of constant support, encouragement, and unfailing outward expressions of love and caring. That from this well-spring of self-esteem I drew the motivation, strength, and, hopefully wisdom, to write *Dying For Compassion*. To say those things would be extreme words of fiction. Wishful thinking to be sure, but, untruths none-the-less.

So, in retrospect, it is not surprising to see that in writing the book I was forced, kicking and screaming, crying and sobbing, back into a battle I thought death had long since wiped from my mind. However, what the mind denies or represses, the heart will not so easily release. Joshua Caliban's efforts to heal his tortured soul stirred exactly the same demons from the muddy waters of my own. Joshua's psychic battles with his dead father staring back at me from my computer began to ring of dialogue encoded in files I thought lost to 'senior moments.'

So, my friends were right. Big deal. I actually came to like the opportunity to, yet again, relive my self-righteous anger and bitterness. To wallow in my self pity. To shout venomous words at 'him' I'd been too afraid to voice when he'd been alive. Once the wound had been lanced, the pus flowed quite freely.

And, as God would have it, underneath the poison there is the core of our beings. A reservoir of unexpressed love. A mother lode of deep golden compassion mixed with a seemingly infinite supply of dark human foibles and imperfections.

However, what came as a total surprise, and a gift of immeasurable and inexpressible proportions, is the fact that as Joshua and his father had their epiphany, so, too, did my father and I.

As Joshua and Martin Caliban came to know, respect, and indeed love one another, 'warts and all', so, too, did Louis Rubin and I. In writing *Dying For Compassion* two relationships of vital importance were, therefore, helped to heal: a father and his son's; and his son's with his own soul. May reading it yield a similar gift for you.

Dying For Compassion is, therefore, proudly dedicated to Louis Rubin, who underneath it all, was a loving, caring, human being doing the best he could with the tools he had.

Acknowledgements

When reading something they themselves have written, particularly when it is something started a long time ago, writers often have the experience of feeling slightly awed; "I can't believe that I actually wrote those words!" The onset of more frequent "senior moments" makes the task of remembering all those who have helped along the way even more daunting.

Many people provided absolutely essential encouragement "never give up, don't quit before the miracle, etc" in the face of a mounting pile of [mostly unopened] rejections from agents. Sincere thanks to Tony Edens, Richard Stone, Vi Zerell, Tom Campbell, Allan London, Reg Graters, Mal Beniston, Paddy Spruce, Kaye Montgomery, Gabrielle Batzer, L J. Lancer, Avery Freed, Deborah Forrest, to name just a few. Members of my own family (Evelyn Neville, Valerie Amoroso, Corey Rubin and Steven Rubin) were equally encouraging. Many others whose names I have forgotten at the moment, were there when I was about to "pack it in". Thank you one and all.

Telling a story is significantly easier than making it an enjoyable and compelling read. When Susan Malone sent me back her editorial suggestions, I had trouble initially seeing the black words from her red markings. But the lessons she taught me turned out to be invaluable, both for my writing [hopefully] and, most assuredly, my humility. And without Tess Black's willingness to take me by the hand, and take Susan's edited manuscript into hers, the needed second draft might never have been born.

When Sarah Fraser, a dear colleague who shares the dream of humanizing healthcare around the globe, saw that draft, she very graciously and enthusiastically opened the door that had heretofore been slammed shut in our faces so many times. Anand Kumar of Kingsham Press wanted to publish it!!

Recognising the need for one more miracle, I approached Tim Boden. Tim was a cyberspace colleague, whom I'd never before met in person, and an accomplished writer in his own right. With all the trepidation of a teenager approaching someone for a first date, I asked Tim if he'd be willing to consider "mid-wifing" my baby through its final stages of birth. You now hold in your hands the results of Tim's generosity, his heart and his skill.

Once a piece of work like *Dying for Compassion* takes a hold of its author's mind, heart and soul, and there are huge blocks of time where everything, and everyone, takes a backseat. So while Tim Boden was *Dying For Compassion*'s editorial mid-wife, Nan Holmes [my soul mate, my friend, my wife] was its emotional mid-wife. Their love and compassion permeates every page. I am truly blessed.

About the Authors

Irwin M. Rubin is an organisational psychologist, President of Temenos Inc. and the author and co-author of several books. T.W. Boden is a writer and healthcare administrator.

Prologue

Chicago, 1985

Joshua straddled the limp body. Palms opened. Fingers splayed. Thump! Thump! He pounded the unmoving man's chest. "Start pumping!" he willed the man's heart.

Breathing heavily, he paused, flexed his fingers, and raked the sweat from his brow up into his tousled, prematurely grey head of hair. He'd been on duty at the hospital for almost thirty-six hours and was nearly exhausted. Seconds later, he resumed, panting with every thrust of his thick, muscular arms.

"Come on, come on, damn it! Don't give up on me yet!"

"It ain't no use, Doc. He's a goner."

Joshua looked up in a daze. How long had André, the night shift orderly, been standing there? Defeated, he braced his massive six-foot-three-inch frame and carefully climbed down from the gurney to prevent the thing rolling haphazardly into the crowded waiting room.

The harsh white light of the emergency room illuminated people sprawled on chairs and huddled in small groups, silently staring back at him. He recognized some of them. There sat Mrs. Katsimbalis, an old woman who still dressed in mourning fifteen years after her husband's death. She came in every Thursday or Friday night, out of loneliness.

Across the aisle, frazzled-looking Mrs. Francetti shook a finger in her son's squalling red face and yanked him upright by a handful of worn shirt. Her abrupt gesture revealed telltale pinholes dotting her arms. Rings of thick, acrid smoke from her cigarette smoldering among the mound of crushed butts in the ashtray hung in the air between mother and son. Caked blood crusted the edges of a nasty-looking gash on the child's head, but Mrs. Francetti had more likely returned to pick up some more tranquilizers.

A few feet away a black man sat by himself, hunched over. Splotches of dried cement flecked his wizened face, twisted with pain. He cradled his arm wrapped in a crude, blood-soaked bandage.

A typical night at Cook County. No sleep, and the countless cups of gray-brown coffee just weren't doing the trick any more. Once, Joshua's residency would have been considered a plum by his medical school colleagues, but that was long ago—before the addicts and the abusers, the blood and death, and the loading dock with its endless supply of broken bodies.

"Doc, there's still someone out there you need to see … another goner."

André again. Joshua sighed wearily. The state, in its infinite wisdom, had passed a requirement that only a physician could pronounce a person dead. The ambulance drivers and morticians quickly figured out that the cheapest and fastest way to find a doctor to sign a certificate was at the County emergency room. A mountain of paperwork grew for everybody.

Joshua reached for his ophthalmoscope—a reflex action.

"You won't be needing it, Doc. Not for this one."

Outside, Joshua filled his lungs with the cool night air. His temples were throbbing. He blinked a few times as he looked up and down the loading dock. Not a hearse or ambulance in sight.

"It ain't on the loading dock." The orderly jerked Joshua around the corner by his arm. "It's over here."

As they rounded the corner, Joshua hesitated almost imperceptibly before his eyes followed the beam of André's flashlight. Something oozed out from under his shoes and his feet slipped. He grabbed the wall to steady himself. After three years of residency, he dreaded what was coming. He gulped the night air, hoping the dread would pass. Finally, he looked down.

"Holy shit! Holy fucking shit!" He was standing in a pool of blood. Within inches of his feet lay the body of a jumper, the pebbled sidewalk surface seemed to be fused with his flattened chest. The blood-soaked plastic I.D. bracelet was unreadable, but still intact. The head looked like a smashed watermelon. The patient's bare legs were covered with warts and lesions.

When he finally controlled his gagging, Joshua placed the ends of his stethoscope into his ears. He moved slowly, disconnected, like a robot.

"Where do you expect to put that thing?" André asked.

Joshua froze, his mouth agape, and then spit out the small amount of vomit that had lodged in his throat. He pressed a fist against his stomach to stem the nausea and then looked up into the blackness of the night. Ten floors above, through an open window, he saw a nurse's face, contorted in horror. Her expression mirrored his own revulsion, even though jumpers were not uncommon here.

And this was not the first AIDS-related suicide at County. Joshua had begged the hospital administration to put bars or screens on the AIDS patients' windows. He could recite their oft-stated excuses from memory: "This is a place of healing—a hospital, not a prison. It would create the wrong image in the community." Sanctimonious bastards. The only thing that mattered to them—he was convinced—was the bottom line.

In the emergency room and in spite of the adrenaline already racing through his blood stream, he reached blindly for a cup of coffee. His shaking hands knocked the coffee clumsily to the floor. He stared listlessly as a cockroach climbed into the cup, came back out, then scurried across the floor, as if to spread the news of its good fortune. Or, Joshua mused cynically, to warn the others of just how bad the coffee was.

A wave of hopelessness washed over him: The best, most up-to-date technology and equipment might help heal diseased bodies, but as long as broken spirits and lost souls were neglected, all their money and effort seemed futile. Good Lord! he thought, unless I happen to be on duty when his file comes down from upstairs, I'll never even know the poor bastard's name.

Joshua's pen hovered over the Cause of Death form as he contemplated what to write. The disease hadn't killed him as much as society's apathy and fear. That same apathy and fear—fueled by greed—kept County's higher-ups from spending a little extra on screens for patients' windows. A jumper at County would hardly command more than a couple paragraphs in an inside section of the newspaper. He was little more than an unfortunate statistic to them—a death waiting to happen, a body taking up space and draining expensive resources. If the truth were told, management might admit the hospital was actually better off with the doomed patient out of the way.

These hated moments occurred way too often. Joshua collected the bile mixed with his saliva onto his tongue and spat into an empty coffee cup. Taking a prescription bottle from his pocket, he held it to the light, momentarily appreciating the shadow-like kaleidoscope shapes created by the capsules of benzedrine shifting against the amber-colored plastic container. Popping the last three remaining pills into his mouth, he snapped his head back, forcing them down dry.

Biting his lower lip, he scrawled, "Nobody gave a shit!" across the Cause of Death form, ripped it off, crumbled it into a ball and dropped it onto the floor. Looking down at his feet, he remembered the hospital's rule to destroy his blood-soaked shoes. We can't protect our patients, but we have plenty infectious-waste rules to protect us from OSHA fines! He seethed with anger, and the pencil in his fingers snapped in half.

"Not in *my* hospital!" he hissed under his breath, "Not when *I'm* in charge!" He flung the broken pencil at the line of roaches marching across his desk.

One

Chicago, 1998

Joshua's Adidas' squeegeed like a dry rubber wiper against glass as he paced the hardwood floor behind his seat in the boardroom. Christ, the air smelled like an empty gymnasium—smelled of the accumulated anxiety running through everyone's blood during the countless meetings held here.

The air conditioning droned in the background, making his head throb. Perhaps the pulsation was merely the drug rushing in his bloodstream. He wasn't normally so sensitive. The machine's low hum merged with the subdued buzzing emanating from his colleagues, talking nervously around the table. Joshua stopped his pacing to stare down at the stark white paper in his hand. The neatly typewritten lines vibrated in front of his eyes. The intestines knotted up deep in his gut—the same as when he looked at a death certificate. Did the words themselves nauseate him, or the nasty shock of dismay when he first saw the memo?

He looked up blankly and scanned the room until he could focus on something, anything at all. His gaze settled on the six foot tall, cylindrical fish tank in the corner to his right. The image of a handsome man in his late forties, distinguished by a full, silver-streaked beard, reflected off the polished glass. Large, but

---

1

well-defined features. Almost aristocratic. He was perversely pleased to see three permanent horizontal lines etched across his forehead, and the skin under his slate grey eyes looked delicate.

The vivid colored tropical fish soothed him for an instant. Ah, to be in that other world—trout fishing on the Root River. But unlike the brute effort of trout fighting to move upstream, these creatures appeared to hang suspended by the slow-motion flutter of gossamer fins, carefully maintaining their individual territories.

Behind the tank, tightly drawn curtains separated the room from the warmth of the setting sun. Usually the curtains were left open. The view of C.C.A.'s atrium across the flowered court-yard three floors below, full of live plants and artwork, calmed Joshua's troubled mind. In the distance, the University of Chicago rose above the horizon like a giant medieval castle. He liked to think that within its chambers the oratory echoing off the walls was one of honest debate.

There wasn't a chance in hell such debate would be heard in this boardroom. In fact, since Joshua had entered the chamber, only Peter Albert had made eye contact with him. Everyone else focused on the long oval conference table in front of them.

Joshua wished he could read their thoughts. The benzedrine pills that he'd popped on his way to the board meeting to flag his waning energies filtered back up. Anger and rage, feelings he hadn't acknowledged in a long time, pushed up from deep inside him to lodge in his throat, leaving a particularly sour taste on his tongue.

He rubbed his temples and closed his eyes, wanting to hit something, to lash out and release the sickness that this betrayal, this cowardly piece of paper, had brought him. But that would be a mistake.

To steady himself, he touched the control panel installed on the table by his chair. Pressing its buttons, he could operate any of the state-of-the-art high-tech equipment with which the room was equipped—the slide projector that receded into the table, the rotating Xerox copier that made perfect replicas of anything placed on its multiple faces. Many times he'd wished the panel included a seat ejection button as well. He would love to send some of the jackasses who occupied the deep leather-and-chrome swivel chairs arranged around the table flying into outer space. A chair scraped on the hardwood floor. How long had he been lost in his own reverie? From the pocket of his starched lab coat he pulled out his reading glasses and positioned them carefully on the bridge of his nose. He peered over the rims at the chit-chatting board members and cleared his throat.

"In case any of you forgot your reading glasses, I'll read this aloud. As *some* of you would know, it's a memo from this Board of Trustees dated June first, 1998 addressed to Damien Rees, Chief Operating Officer," Joshua said, not even trying to mask his sarcasm.

"'A special meeting was held by the Board of Trustees to discuss a situation at Care Corporation of America that we feel has reached crisis proportions. Morale has become so poor that several of our younger, better-trained doctors are threatening to leave. In fact, we've discovered that some are currently interviewing for positions with our competitors. We believe the precipitating factor has been the unexpectedly poor financial performance presented by operations this past year.'"

He looked up at the group and let the silence of his pause hang heavily for a moment, then continued, "'We all agree that these are tough times and that it is vital that our doctors believe that we are looking out for their interests. Unfortunately, in recent months, it has come to our attention that our doctors increasingly mistrust your judgment. Further alienation will create the risk of losing more good people, and thereby threatens the future of the organization. Growth without quality

---

3

physicians on the staff is impossible. Without a change in leadership, our ability to attract and hold the finest of care providers will be seriously undermined.'

"'After careful consideration, the Board has decided it is in the best interests of patient care that we ask you to submit your resignation as Chief Operating Officer. In light of your long years of service, we realize that this will be a difficult decision for you to accept. We acknowledge that you have contributed to our past successes, but change is necessary to allow us to move forward. We are certain that a satisfactory severance package can be put together to meet your needs.'"

Joshua took off his glasses, folded them, and put them back in his coat pocket. He rose, glanced again at the memo, then dropped it back onto the table. Very deliberately, he stared at each of the men. He could feel the color rising in his face, but his resolve was as hard and cold as ice.

Paul Blake, the hospital's chief anesthesiologist, glared back defiantly through deeply set eyes but soon looked away.

Roger Rosen, a fellow surgeon, averted Joshua's gaze, his pancake-like face flushed. Roger was one of Joshua's medical school classmates and headed one of the most successful—and productive—cardiac transplant and bypass teams in the country. When he wasn't indulging in his other primary passion, sailing on the lake, he and his five-person team could give new life to as many as four patients and their families in a single day, adding six figures to Care Corporation's bottom line in the process. Hopefully Roger had simply succumbed to a bad wind and got caught up in the cabal that had produced the shameful memo. Surely he wouldn't be the one to lead such an insurrection.

Next sat Scott MacDonald, proctologist and chief of internal medicine and recognized jackass of the lot. Nah, too much of a fool to have been the instigator. At the moment, his balding head sported a furrowed brow. No doubt he was at least among the abettors. Scott was a bandwagon jumper.

Continuing around the table, Joshua's anger softened as he looked at Ross Benson, the chief of pathology. Ross was such a class act, his reputation for fairness so solid, that Joshua had appointed him head of the Mortality Committee. No committee was more feared and respected by the doctors at C.C.A., because in a malpractice case, it was Ross who would judge if a fellow physician could have prevented a patient's death. In a single instant, Ross had the power to wipe away a lifetime of work and bring a man's reputation to utter ruin, or to save him from destruction. Now the pathologist awkwardly examined his perfectly manicured hands—a customary gesture that seemed to Joshua as if he were seeking to rid them of the perpetual smell of death.

Finally, saving his best hope for last, Joshua met Peter Albert's steady gaze. The hint of dismay in his hazel eyes indicated that he hadn't known of the memo either.

Getting a grip, Joshua reached down and fingered the memo again, thoughtfully running his tongue over his lips. Indeed, it was real. Without speaking, he started a slow circuit around the table. The heavy silence of the room was broken only by his squeaking shoes and crackling starched whites. He stopped behind Paul Blake and dropped both his hands onto the anesthesiologist's Ichabod Crane-like bony shoulders. Joshua's sensitive fingers, trained by years of delicate surgical procedures, could register the slightest shift in the man's heartbeat or his breathing. With his right hand, he took Blake's copy of the memo and held it closer. Same memo. He crushed it into a little ball and let it fall back onto the burnished oak table.

Joshua repeated this performance with Roger and was halfway around the table when Jane Sherwood arrived and slid into her regular place at the right of Joshua's seat. Jane, C.C.A.'s corporate attorney, had graduated second in her class at Harvard Law School. She could have had her pick of higher-paying jobs, but she'd chosen to work with Joshua because she was attracted to the healing arts. Joshua had never doubted her commitment and was greatly relieved to see her. But why the tardiness? He gave her a nod.

When he'd gone around the entire room and settled back into his chair, Joshua broke his silence. "I assume, gentlemen, that some of you thought today was April Fool's Day, and that this is your idea of a joke."

He pushed his copy of the memo to Jane to read. Her robin blue eyes scanned it with a radar-like precision developed from years of pouring over lengthy briefs, while at the same time gauging the tension in the room. She stole a look at Scott MacDonald, seated on Joshua's left.

Although her Barbie-doll face betrayed nothing, Joshua was sure he knew what was on her mind. She had told him once that Scott's body reminded her of the stick figures kids drew, with matchstick legs protruding from a beer-barrel belly. His head sat askew on top of his shoulders as if his neck had been broken— something a lot of people would love to have done. Even Jane had admitted sharing that fantasy on occasion. Always interrupting conversations, he would then stumble over himself as he tried to get his words out. A real pest. Scott was just one of those people you loved to hate.

Scott's bug eyes darted nervously around the room. "This isn't a joke, Joshua. We're serious," he mumbled.

"You can bet your sweet ass it isn't, Scott," Joshua said, leaning forward and pointing a menacing finger. A ripple of anxious laughter followed. "I don't consider it a joke at all that this board would dare to hold meetings and draft a memo like this behind my back, ostensibly to have been authored by me! So perhaps you'd like to lead off with an explanation of what the hell you guys are trying to pull." Joshua leaned back and waited.

Scott squirmed before stammering, "We're very concerned with the erosion of morale. We felt it was our responsibility to act on behalf of the organization."

"Who is this *'we,'* Scott?" Joshua asked. "Who among you have decided it's in the best interest of patient care that Damien be asked to submit his resignation?"

Scott floundered like a drowning rat, looking helplessly around the room until his gaze met Ross Benson's.

In a metronomic tone, Ross began, "Look, Joshua, the subgroup who prepared the memo probably should've talked to you first." He abandoned his nails and ran his hands once through his thick, immaculately combed silver-grey hair. "But we felt the situation was getting very serious and it was urgent that something be done."

"I don't doubt your *commitment*," Joshua replied. "And I know better than anyone else that our situation is serious. Otherwise I'd never have agreed to hold this closed meeting. But I'll *not* tolerate sandbagging of someone who's not here to defend himself. If that's clear to everyone, we can proceed."

Joshua's breathing had returned to normal. Clearly, he had an enemy close by. Time would yield the guilty party. But for now, the moment had passed, and it was business as usual.

Roger Rosen leaned forward. "Let's face it, the cash cows have had their teats caught in a wringer. None of us became a doctor with the expectation of working for a large organization. Like it or not, that's the way it is, and that's the way it's going to be. But I didn't claw my way through Harvard and bust my chops in residency just to have some tight-ass bean counter tell me how to practice medicine." Roger sat back, the corners of his lips arching slightly toward the ends of his pencil-thin mustache.

Joshua cocked his head. "I understand your feelings, but Damien isn't telling you how to practice surgery."

"The *hell* he isn't," Roger barked. "He's telling me I've got to do more, get paid less, and forget about my retirement savings. What does he know about cutting open people's hearts? The only thing he knows about cutting is expenses, including our salaries."

Joshua jolted upright and pulled at his beard. "I see your point, but that's not his job. He's supposed to watch over the health of the whole organization. Do you honestly feel you could step into *his* shoes?" Joshua paused. Hopefully the bitching wouldn't escalate into a pitched battle.

"Damien works for *me*, not the other way around," Scott blurted, wiping the beads of sweat forming on his balding pate with the back of his hand. "Talk about the tail wagging the dog. He throws me a bone and tells me the cupboard is bare."

Peter flexed his shoulders and cleared his throat. "The point, gentlemen, is that we *all* work for C.C.A., and C.C.A. works for its patients. Some of you guys are suffering from early Alzheimer's. This isn't the first cash flow problem we've ever had. Remember a few years back, when we had a similar financial crisis? It was Damien who convinced us to invest in a new computer billing system. That alone cut our accounts receivable delay in half. He even figured out a way to recoup some of the massive collectibles we had outstanding from the heavy bleeders."

God bless Peter. No wonder Joshua loved the man who would someday occupy his seat.

"True enough," Ross agreed, his measured tone raising an octave. "We'd never have pulled through the last couple of years, what with the deluge of AIDS patients we've had storming the gates."

"Yeah, but we funded that new computer out of our operating capital." Scott's pudgy arms were waving uncontrollably, fluttering away from his barrel body like a burst balloon through the air. "My wife is going to scream bloody murder if I tell her I've agreed to take a cut in pay."

Joshua grimaced. But he also had some sympathy for Scott's feelings. He firmly believed his team deserved their salaries. Money was little enough reward for the kind of nerve required to look death in the face, day after day. But money was like any other addiction. The more you had, the more you craved. And some of these men here—and their wives—had well-established habits.

"Both Peter and I have studied Damien's proposals very carefully," Joshua said. "The painful fact is that—even if we decided *together* at some point in the future that a restructuring was in the best interests of patient care—we can't avoid biting the bullet this year."

Ross touched his fingers together making an arch. "Can't we borrow some money from the bank?"

Ah, Ross was coming around. Joshua shook his head. "No, we can't. Every time we increase our line of credit these days, the bank takes another pound of flesh. Our last building campaign strengthened our market position dramatically, but left us leveraged to the hilt."

All the doctors except Paul nodded. Each had personally co-signed the bank notes and knew what kind of figures Joshua was talking about.

Peter leaned back, locked his fingers together over his head, and cracked his knuckles. "So, Joshua, can you tell us what you plan to do about the board's concerns?"

"I'll speak with Damien privately and make certain we've explored every option for easing the pressure. And I'll respect the group's wishes to keep the details of this meeting private."

Joshua looked around the table and folded his hands together. They still trembled with anger. The pills weren't serving him well.

"And just so there's no confusion, I expect never again to be *surprised* by a typed memo sitting in front of my chair awaiting my signature. For all our sakes, I hope Damien doesn't get wind of this before I have a chance to speak to him. Furthermore, I will honor what I assume your expectations are regarding my discussion with Damien. I'll give you the results in another session, without his attendance. And that, gentlemen, will be the last closed meeting this board will conduct. I presume there's no further business."

Joshua glanced around the table briefly. Then he rose, turned, and headed out the door and down the hall. An uneasy feeling churned in the pit of his stomach. He hoped another pill would help him stay on top of things.

As Joshua's broad back disappeared through the boardroom door, Paul Blake's gaze shifted to his fellow board members. Peter moved to intercept Jane before she could leave the room. "Birds of a feather," Paul smirked. They'd no doubt be chirping in Joshua's ear before the rest of them were out of the building. And as far as Ross, Roger, and Scott were concerned—what a bunch of gutless losers, like rats deserting a sinking ship.

Paul raised his arm in a Gestapo-like salute that halted them in their tracks. "Meet me at the restaurant," he said, leaving no room for quarrel. "You may be anxious to get home to your families, but we have to debrief tonight."

Paul had chosen not to speak during the meeting. He could tell from the beginning that the momentum wasn't going to go their way, and he wanted to observe everything with careful attention, stowing away all the minute details of what everyone did and said. Now, he hurried through the hall to the elevator, then to the parking lot. He wanted a cigarette that badly. And, if he got there fast enough, he might even have time to enjoy a few precious drops of something more heavenly than smoke.

Pulling out of C.C.A.'s parking lot, he gunned the engine. With an agonized squeal, the rear wheels propelled his fire-engine red Porsche onto the entrance of the expressway. The car fishtailed into the right lane, trailing an acrid cloud of black exhaust smoke. But a few seconds later he was brought to a screeching halt, stuck behind a solid wall of rush hour traffic. In a sweat, breathing heavily, he stared at his hands gripping the steering wheel, his knuckles white. He deliberately relaxed them and tried to slow his breathing.

God, how he hated Joshua Caliban! A few years ago, Paul was the anesthesiologist on Joshua's O.R. team. The patient, an elderly woman, wasn't responding to the transfusion. Kathy Marshall, Joshua's favorite O.R. nurse, spotted the problem. The IV petcock valve was clogged.

Paul should have checked it himself. But since he had not been scheduled for surgery that day, Paul's mind was where his body should have been—in bed with Scott MacDonald's wife, Elaine. Ah, the delights of Elaine's thighs and what lay between them—her most appealing attribute. Joshua blew up. "If you would get your head out of your ass, Doctor, we might be able to keep this patient alive."

Their patient didn't die. She didn't even suffer any damage. At first, Paul considered himself lucky, then dismissed his culpability. Joshua not only had embarrassed him, but he'd done so in front of the O.R. staff. Then he added to the humiliation by refusing to work with him for the better part of a year. Long ago—after his father had teased him about the size of his penis in front of his friends—Paul resolved never to allow anyone to shame him again without paying for it.

Dr. Joshua Caliban, holier-than-thou, fighting to bring healing to the suffering masses with his lectures about "cradle-to-the-grave" care. One would think he was Jesus Christ Himself. He lived to bring Joshua down, to humiliate him like Joshua had done to him, and to top it off by taking his throne—becoming head of C.C.A. himself.

In spite of himself though, he had to admit admiring Joshua's self-control in the boardroom tonight. His response to the coup was calculated, unflinching, and powerful.

The traffic began to flow and Paul eased up on the brake. But, Good Lord! Scott MacDonald was *pathetic* compared to Joshua. What a piece of work. He had actually been Paul's first recruit, mostly because he'd been so easy. Elaine was the key to her husband. She could manipulate him with sex, precisely because she despised him.

Of course, sex was also the key to Elaine. He cultivated her needs, teasing her with clandestine meetings. Although not his first choice for these sexual indulgences, Elaine was both willing and available. If he could get information out of her, all the better. She told Paul all about Scott's predilections in the bedroom, how he loved it when she'd make him beg and then reward him with a "golden shower." She fanned the fires of Scott's passions while she inflamed his naturally paranoid nature with allegations against his colleagues—allegations planted in her brain by Paul.

Once he had Scott, Paul targeted Ross. Because of his friendship with Joshua, he'd been the hardest to recruit. But in the end, Paul used that friendship to sway the "nail man," as he called the chief of pathology. The nickname was a dig at Ross' regular role in nailing coffins shut with his pathology reports. After all, Joshua was forever urging his executives to act on their own

---

12

initiative. It was a good stratagem, but after tonight's meeting, Paul knew he couldn't count on Ross' support.

Then there was Roger, whose natural distrust was easily transferred to Damien. It wasn't personal. All bean counters were the same, as far as Roger was concerned. The Rosen family's medical roots went back three generations—a hundred years of Rosen men fending for themselves in private practice. That is, until Roger's generation. And even though the changed marketplace now made opening his own practice unrealistic, Roger took it as a personal failure. Plus, he had four daughters to support.

Because of Roger's normally unruffled demeanor, manipulating him into being the one to suggest the idea of replacing Damien was a snap. Sounding like they were his own thoughts, Roger had convinced Ross that the growing mistrust among the troops might best be resolved by installing a medical doctor—one of their own as Chief Operating Officer.

Paul exited the twelve-lane thoroughfare. He had made good time, in spite of the traffic, and he would have a few moments to himself. He was skilled at finding out-of-the-way meeting places for all his activities. Paul liked to think he was, in his own way, continuing the tradition of Edward III who originated the strategy of holding unauthorized councils of concerned members of the king's court. Edward held his meetings deep in the castle's basement, like the room where they'd been meeting. It was a windowless chamber lined with rows of aging wines. Painted stars on the ceilings gave the illusion that the conspirators were operating under the sanction of the heavens. Their objectives weren't nearly as admirable as his.

He pulled into the restaurant's parking lot and chose a secluded space at the back. Reaching for his car phone, he dialed and three rings later Damien's familiar recorder said, "I can't

---

come to the phone right now. Leave a message of any length you wish."

Disliking answering machines, Paul considered hanging up. Only the devil knew who listened to one's messages, and one could hardly deny anything committed to tape. But what the hell? He laughed aloud, flashing back on a wonderfully erotic afternoon he and Damien had spent together. Pleading his need for a sports fix, he managed to get one day away from Elaine.

They had watched the now-famous Denver-Cleveland AFC Championship game on TV. With only seconds to play, his team behind, and the entire length of the field to cover, John Elway knelt in the huddle to motivate his troops. Paul and Damien imagined Elway enthusiastically telling his teammates, "We've got them just where we want them!" It was a famous quote of his. Elway then marched his team to victory against seemingly insurmountable odds.

"This is John Elway calling," Paul spoke into the receiver. "I've just come from a closed huddle. We penetrated their red zone but we weren't able to ram it in. But we gained some good yardage. We've got them just where we want them. All we have to do is keep coming at them—hard. More … first thing tomorrow."

Paul smiled. Good lines to remember.

Satisfied there was no one around, he rolled up his sleeve and snapped on the rubber strap. A vein popped up instantly. Before he could count to ten, the ice-cold tip of the syringe delivered the exquisite relief of the acid he so loved. God was surely looking out for him, he thought with smug satisfaction.

Now all he had to do was make sure motor-mouth MacDonald and the rest of his star chambers crew didn't run to tell Damien what had happened tonight.

14

Two

The walk back to his office was longer through the underground maze that served as C.C.A.'s basement, but Joshua needed a few minutes to settle the angry waves reverberating through his brain. If he had come face-to-face with Paul, the consequences might have been ugly.

How could his dreams in residency about his own hospital turn so easily into nightmares? He was often lost in a sad review of how he'd gotten into this mess in the first place.

During the board meeting, an involuntary shudder had jolted him as he looked down at the document awaiting his signature. His mother's face rose up every time he lifted a pen to sign his full name with its hard-won title: Joshua Nathan Caliban, *M.D.* If not for her, he would never have become a doctor of medicine. In fact, he probably would never have become interested in any kind of healing.

Stopping in front of the water fountain just outside the morgue, he visualized a few faces he wouldn't mind seeing on the slabs inside. He let the cold water splash across his lips and swallowed a mouthful, then closed his eyes, hoping the pressure he felt might lessen. When that failed, he flexed his shoulders, rubbed the back of his neck, and rolled his head a few times, listening to the crunching of the vertebrae. The ache in his neck inevitably heralded mental reruns of life-draining memories of his father, Martin Caliban.

⤜⟋⤛

Martin was dark and medium-built, stocky and muscular in the arms and torso and short in the legs. He'd been bald from his early twenties; the skin that stretched over his rounded skull freckled lightly from the hours he spent out in the sun on his car lot. He had a boxer's pugilistic stance: solid and rooted on his feet. His arms and shoulders commanded great strength, lashing out in vicious, stabbing jabs at anything that got in his way. Ironically, he had beautiful hands. They had gotten him through the Depression working as a milliner until he had scraped together enough to go into business for himself. This one scrap of sensitivity was what Joshua clung to whenever Martin's temper escalated to blind rage—which was whenever things didn't go the way he planned. Packed into his father's stocky, muscular frame was more meanness, determination and narrow-minded intelligence than you'd find in the finest pure-bred pit bull.

Joshua had the misfortune to have shot up a full foot taller than his father by the time he was sixteen. "Don't think that just because your feet are bigger than mine, you're gonna find it easy to fill my shoes!" Martin would say to him. "You'll be looking up to me all of your life."

And it was true: For the rest of his father's life, Joshua seemed to deliberately shrink down to his father's expectations. Accepting his size as a fault, he drew up his broad shoulders and slouched. But the only result was chronic pain between his shoulder blades, a condition that flared into a full-blown migraine and a stiff neck when he was under severe stress.

Martin always dreamed of the day his only son would take over the car dealership he'd built from nothing. And that dream hung like a concrete block around Joshua's aching neck.

On his seventeenth birthday, Martin told him, "I know you're smart enough to know how to make babies. Let me tell you something even more valuable. You build a business the same way you grow a family—one good fuck at a time."

Joshua didn't dare ask out loud the question that popped into his mind: So why am I an only child? He never did develop the nerve to ask his father. He didn't have to. As Joshua grew into adulthood, it became clear that the only things Martin Caliban loved in life were business and fishing.

On the day his mother died, the same day he was to have graduated from college, Joshua knew with absolute certainty he would never follow in his father's footsteps.

Naomi Caliban had undergone a partial mastectomy to combat breast cancer the year before. All seemed well after the operation—except for the headaches. But that was nothing new; she'd suffered from headaches and depression as long as Joshua could remember.

Martin paid no attention. In his view, Naomi's headaches were only a woman's excuse for not servicing her husband, although he was careful never to say that to her face. Besides, he was rarely home anyway. His life was on the lot, pushing cars, pulling himself out of the poverty he had grown up with and so feared.

But Joshua devoted himself to his mother's care, partly in defiance of his father's attitude and partly because he craved Naomi's softness. He spent hours sitting with her on the edge of her bed. They played Scrabble or did crossword puzzles. Sometimes, he massaged his mother's feet or her back to ease her discomfort. She told him he had magic hands.

⁓⟋⟍⁓

Joshua's reverie was interrupted by a hallway intersection demanding a decision: The path leading toward the parking lot was the least direct route to his office. The other would bring him through the hospital kitchen, a beehive of activity at this hour when several hundred hospital dinners would be rolling off the assembly line. Joshua decided to take the long way through the parking lot. He punctuated his resolve by locking his fingers together and bending them back to crack his knuckles. As the popping sound softly echoed down the empty gray tunnel before him, he could almost here his mother whispering her oft-repeated advice: "Follow your intuition."

⁂

Naomi had been the only source of warmth, beauty, and mystery in Joshua's life, and Martin treated her with ill-concealed disdain. "Take some more of those damn pills the doctor gave you. I pay an arm and a leg for them."

One terrifying night she screamed from her room, "They're not working anymore!" And Martin finally agreed to take her to see a new specialist.

On the way to the doctor's office, his father launched into one of his favorite tirades. "Your mother's illness is all in her head. Her doctor says he can't find nothin' wrong, but he doesn't have the kind of X-ray equipment they have at Mayo. So he sends us over there, like these guys think I don't know about padding bills, about kissing each other's ass. And right in the middle of the holidays with the new models due on the lot any day."

Joshua had glared at the back of his father's billiard ball head, wishing he had the guts to tell him to shut up. When they returned from that visit, Joshua was surprised to see how shaken his father was. Martin wore the grim, ashen color of a man who'd seen his own death. He went right to bed without so much as a word to go with the forlorn hug and kiss he'd given Joshua. But that kiss betrayed him. Martin Caliban was so rarely affectionate.

Two months later, his mother was admitted to the hospital for the last time. Joshua was in his senior year of mechanical engineering, the program his father had selected for him. He visited his mother as often as he could, and tried to drown his pain in the bottom of a bottle—a habit he had taken up in school.

For the last two months of her life, Naomi was in a coma, except for those occasions when Joshua came to see her.

"It's quite amazing," the nurses reported. "She opens her eyes the minute you set foot in the lobby of the hospital. And she closes them again the minute you leave."

Even now, in the midst of a sea of cars parked underneath the hospital of his dreams, Joshua still felt this psychic connection with his mother. For a moment, it helped ease the awful loneliness. He leaned against the fender of a nearby car and shut his eyes. Would the tears ever dry up?

One night the doctor told them there was nothing more he could do for Naomi.

"What do you mean, nothing?" Joshua cried out. But all of his bravado and his demanding posture dropped away as quickly as it had appeared. His lip quivered uncontrollably. "This is a big hospital, the best hospital. You're her doctor and she's dying."

The doctor had continued in a monotone, "If you wish, I'll order the removal of her intravenous feeding tubes, but I'll continue to sedate her so she'll feel as little discomfort as possible."

The room had spun in silence for an eternity. Martin Caliban just sat staring out into space. At last he rose slowly and stumbled toward the door. He pulled the door shut behind him, his parting words hanging in the air like the caption from a cartoon picture not yet drawn. "My son can decide what to do."

Still staring at the closed door, Joshua whispered, "Stop feeding my mother."

Joshua took the night vigil. At five-thirty the next morning, Joshua lifted his mother's seventy pound body from the bed on which she had lain for the past few months. He did so slowly, delicately, afraid that her wrinkled, cold skin would peel off in his arms. As he cradled the diminished body, Naomi's eyes opened. A tear ran down his cheek and fell onto her cracked, parched lips. Her tongue, scaled with the white bumps of death, licked at the moisture instinctively.

"I'll be okay, Mama. I'll be okay. You don't need to worry about protecting me from Dad anymore. I'm a big boy now. I can take care of myself. Go to sleep now, Mama. Sweet dreams." He kissed each of her eyes, and Naomi Caliban closed them for the last time.

Martin Caliban came staggering downstairs in a drunken stupor just as Joshua opened the front door. "Mom's dead," he said. His father convulsed with a sob and buried his unshaven, ashen face in his dinner-plate-sized hands. It was only the thinnest taste of the loneliness that would follow Martin the rest of his years, but Joshua had no more pity left for his father—he felt no sorrow.

After the funeral he informed his father that he'd decided to apply to medical school. His courage was bolstered by a firm promise to himself: He would *never again* feel dependent or helpless. That determination locked in his heart became the driving force behind his continuing success.

The chug-chug of the security guard's go-cart sputtering to a stop snapped Joshua back to reality. "Are you okay, Dr. Caliban? Are you okay, sir?"

Joshua swallowed hard and rubbed a tear out of the corner of his eye before he responded, "Fine, thanks. Just a little dirt in my lenses, that's all. Thanks for checking, though."

Feeling self-conscious, he ducked into the elevator and pushed the UP button several times. The bottle of pills in the bottom drawer of his desk beckoned loudly through the fog of painful memories swirling in his head.

Joshua was halfway through his outer office before he realized Mary Howard was still there putting on her coat. She had been his first nurse. When he discovered her natural aptitude for numbers—a skill she attributed to being forced to fend for herself after her husband's untimely death—he prevailed upon her to give up nursing and become his Executive Secretary. Mary knew him as well as his wife did and was just as loyal and loving. Her uncanny ability to know what was going on in C.C.A. ofttimes caught him off-balance.

Joshua put his hands on his hips. "How many times have I told you not—"

Mary held her hand in the air. "I know, I know! Not to catch your workaholism. I'm outta here."

"Jane's on her way up," he barked as she moved past him. "Don't lock the downstairs door."

"Got it. See you tomorrow. Looks like it's goin' to be a stormy day."

Joshua sat down at his desk and shook his head. The tone of his own voice rang in his ears and sparked a twinge of guilt. He was rarely that abrupt with Mary, and when he was, he knew it meant that stress had pushed his temper to the flashpoint. He opened his bottom desk drawer. What could he take that would level these damn mood swings? But before he could check his stash, he heard Jane's high-heeled footsteps.

"Knock, knock!" she called as the carpeting silenced her heels. She didn't try to hide her amazement as she sauntered into his office: "Some bloodbath!"

Rolling his head from side to side to try and relieve the tension he felt, Joshua observed, "The board is getting harder to handle."

"That's what I want to talk to you about," Jane said. "I know it's late and you've had a long day, but this'll only take a minute. I heard a consultant speak the other day—an organizational psychologist."

"Oh, great, you think our situation calls for a second opinion?" Joshua regretted his sharp reply immediately. "Look Jane, I'm already married to a therapist, and, as a matter of fact, I'd like to get home to see her. Ruth's been away all week."

As if approaching the bench, Jane put her hands on the edge of Joshua's desk. "This woman isn't a personal shrink. She's a corporate psychologist. Dr. Moerae King. I've checked her out and her credentials are impressive. She got her PhD right here at the University of Chicago."

Joshua pulled at the end of his beard. "Come on, Jane! You know how busy I am—*and* the financial pressure we're under. I can't be wasting time or money talking to some academic who's never had to meet a payroll."

"Her clients include the CEOs of several top Fortune 500 companies. She's got personal references from Kaiser and Mayo. Please, just meet her."

Joshua smiled in spite of himself. Jane was skilled at playing to both judge and jury and always in that same measured tone. The mention of Kaiser and Mayo were calculated to break down his resistance. If the big guns could accept outside help, then why couldn't he?

Joshua sighed and leaned back. "How much is this escapade going to cost us?"

"Her first consultation is free. If you both decide to proceed, then she would continue on a retainer." Her sparkling robin's-egg blue eyes stared evenly at him. "She's not interested in any one-night stand."

"You mean she's either cocky or independently wealthy."

"Quite the contrary. Dr. King is a woman on a mission."

Joshua bit his lower lip and leaned forward. "Come on, Jane, don't you think we can handle this on our own? If I need anyone, it's a financial wizard who can tell me how to get the board off my back *without* cutting the doctors' salaries by ten percent. But a corporate shrink?"

Jane shook her head hard. Pushing her red flop of hair back into place, she took precise aim and delivered a perfect shot: "Exactly! For instance, how much of your *own* surgery time has been taken up in the last six months fighting fires and trying to cope with your board?"

She knew how much he preferred being a doctor over running his hospital. A little more subdued, he responded, "Objection overruled, counselor. Proceed."

Jane released her grip on the desk and sat down. "Dr. King gave a speech the other day at the American Bar Association luncheon I attended. She made two points that impressed me: One, she said that organizations act just like human beings, simply because they're made up of human beings. And, like people, organizations go through all the same stages of growing up—like the terrible twos, the tantrums and rebellions, all those obnoxious infantile and adolescent behaviors that drove our parents nuts." Jane grinned at him.

"We've got a bunch of self-centered, snot-nosed teenagers on our hands, is that your point?"

"I rest my case." She folded her delicate hands and leaned back in her chair.

"Okay, okay. What was the second point that impressed you?"

"What I just told you was the good news. The bad news, according to Dr. King, is that children won't grow up whole and healthy unless the parents who are raising them change their own behavior first. Our leading physicians—the board—conduct themselves in the operating room similarly to how they behave and make decisions in the boardroom."

Joshua sat upright and snapped his fingers. "Exactly! The *board* is the problem!"

Jane pursed her unmade-up lips and paused. "With all due respect, Joshua, they're just one part of the problem. And they'll continue to be a problem until *their* parent, their father—"

"Their chairman, you mean." Interrupted Joshua as he tapped his chest. He neither needed, nor tolerated having his nose rubbed in the obvious.

His exhausted sigh declared her victory, and his tone was subdued as he said, "All right, Jane, you win. But right now the only shrink I'm anxious to see is Ruth. Is there anything else I need to know about Dr. King before I call her?"

"Hmmm. Let's see: Well, Marital status single … and, oh yes, you're already scheduled to meet her at ten tomorrow morning. You have luncheon reservations at La Boheme."

Joshua marveled at Jane's confidence that he would give in to her suggestion. But he nodded his approval. "I'm glad to see that you, at least, don't have to be told how to do your job," he said, smiling. "And as always, I appreciate your initiative more than I can say."

C.C.A.'s corporate attorney grabbed her briefcase, stood up and put a supportive hand on Joshua's shoulder. "Say hello to Ruth for me and ask her to give me a buzz when she has time for lunch."

Joshua sat alone in the silence long after Jane left, his thoughts far away in the mountains. If he could just get away for a while and stand waist-deep in the freezing water, peering at the trout

---

hiding in the rocks' shadows. The rushing water would drown out the incessant chatter cluttering the background of his mind.

But the battle raging with the board made his stomach queasy, hot, and tense. What shocked him most was his failure to judge how critical the situation had become. How could he have been so unaware of the growing discontent of the doctors? Had *he* misjudged Damien so badly?

C.C.A. had started out as a well-run, modest-sized practice that had grown into the fifth largest health care organization in the country. Sure, he was still the majority stockholder, but he could never again wield the power he'd held in the early days, and he missed his nearly total control. Damn this challenge to his authority!

"God, I hate this constant fucking pressure," he said out loud. He wanted a drink. But even more, he wanted to see Ruth and run his fingers through her hair. He loved to play with her pony-tail that always shined like a thoroughbred's well-brushed coat. Hoping to God that she was already on her way home, he would rather drown in the comforts of her body than in the bottle of Jack Daniels stashed in his office cabinet.

The phone rang, stinging his nerves like a pistol shot. Please be Ruth.

"Hi, sweetheart, it's me." Her soft voice eased the pressure.

"Who's me?" he asked.

"How many women call you on your private line to say, 'Hi, sweetheart?'"

"Would you promise to hold it against me if I told you the truth?" Joshua teased.

"So how has my handsome fixer of broken hearts been doing while I'm away?"

"Let's see." He counted on his fingers. "There were three plumbing repairs, five engine overhauls, and two galling carbu-retors. And how's my emotional garbage collector been doing?"

"Never has that epithet been more apt. You know what a conference of therapists is like—two papers on shitty anal fixations, one classically electrifying complex with a few Oedipal chasers, and untold numbers of mental jerk-offs. Still, I managed to avoid letting even the most aggressive of them drag me off to his couch."

"How do you do that?"

"Do what?" The lilt in her voice sounded like music. "Know what I'm thinking," he answered softly.

"It's really easy, sweetheart. You have such a one-track mind."

"I'd like to think of myself as a specialist, thank you very much, rather than a man with a one-track mind. But, Ruth," he said, a serious edge coming into his voice, "I can't ever be sure, after what I did to you a few years ago. You know I'd never look at another woman again—"

"I do know that, Joshua," Ruth replied. "I also know you must be feeling really stretched."

"I just miss you, honey. It's been a hellish week."

Ruth's voice grew softer. "So tell me about it."

"I'd rather wait until I see you. When are you getting in?"

"That's why I'm calling. My flight's been delayed until tomorrow morning. The weather has tied up all the outgoing flights and I'm afraid I'll be spending the night in a cheerless hotel room. I'm sorry, Joshua."

Joshua slumped in his chair, the telephone gripped tightly in his hand.

"Oh, well, where do I start?" He tugged at his beard and bit his lip, fighting the tears of disappointment that had sprung unbidden to his eyes. "It all came to a head tonight. With one exception, the board surprised the hell out of me by calling an urgent, unscheduled meeting. The upshot of it is that they're really pissed about C.C.A.'s financial situation. Damien's insisting that all of us take a ten percent pay cut. And the board is acting as though he had told them their mothers were being raped and their homes pillaged." He sighed deeply and paused. "You know, Ruth, the same old shit."

"I'll be on the first plane out of here in the morning, darling, and go straight home. After a quick look at the mail and a nap, I'll be raring to go when you get home. How's that sound?"

"Like the best offer I'm going to get. I love you."

Joshua held the receiver until Ruth had hung up. Then he slammed it down and leaned back in his chair, rested his hands on his belly and stared at the wedding picture on his desk.

～⌒∽⌒～

If he hadn't taken Psych 101 in med school, he'd have never met Ruth Jacobs. He had been in control of every romantic relationship in his life. But it became clear from the start that their decisions would be jointly made or they simply would not remain together. And they both wanted very much to be together.

A stunning beauty by any standards, Joshua found Ruth especially irresistible. She resembled his mother in so many ways. Like his mother, Ruth had long flowing hair that flopped in front of her right eye when she tilted her head, the deep russet locks flickering like firelight on a hearth. Her body was lush, rounded and full. Her heavy breasts and wide hips resembled one of the earth goddess votives she kept on her office bookcase. The warmth of her creamy skin gave off its own exuberant perfume that Joshua loved to inhale. A sweet cream scented houri, she was the embodiment of all the unfulfilled dreams of his youth. But Ruth was very clear that she would never be Joshua's mother.

Her openness, awareness and courage floored him more than their chemistry. She had told him on their second date that becoming a psychologist and paying her own tuition in spite of having wealthy parents was her way to heal the scars etched in her soul by an abusive childhood. Oh, that he could talk so openly about his childhood.

⟲⟳

Joshua rubbed his throbbing temples. The pressure on his head felt like a vise. He wouldn't go home tonight. The traffic was more than he could bear. He would sleep instead on the daybed in his office.

He showered in his private bathroom, toweled off, dropped two red halcyon into his mouth and swallowed them dry. Hopefully tonight the little red ones would do their work without subjecting him to those intensely disturbing dreams and flashbacks that seemed to occur more and more frequently.

He hated not being able to control them, never knowing if he'd have to endure them even before he was blessed with sleep. He stumbled to the daybed, threw his head on the pillow, and fell into a dark and troubled sleep.

⟲⟳

"Chulah, chulah, kill, kill." The words roared through young Joshua's ears. Thousands of fans in the fronton were screaming at the top of their lungs at the jai alai players to drive the pelota into the crack in the corner of the front wall. If they succeeded, the baseball-shaped pelota would drop to the floor like a duck full of buckshot, ending of the game for the opposing team.

The sound echoed off the walls behind them and receded as Joshua and his father walked toward the betting windows. Joshua was old enough now to bet by himself, and the thrill of playing his own hunches added to his love of the game. But he kept his intuitions secret. Martin Caliban thought hunches were a waste of time. He spent hours studying the players and their histories to develop his strategy, making his bets with the assurance that only practical, hardheaded logic was driving his selection.

"What are you throwing your money away on this time?" Martin asked him.

"I think I'll stay with my birthday, two-four-six. And Mama wants me to play our address again for her, five-six-eight."

Martin's full lips puckered and his bushy eyebrows peaked. "Both of you are too sentimental. Your mother's got a naturally bleeding heart and a soft head. It'll cost us a fortune. The eight team couldn't get laid in a cathouse, and by the time the five and six get up, they'll already be behind."

"You wanna book the bet yourself?" Joshua dared to say.

"Listen to this. My son, the bookmaker! Yeah, I'll book the bet and I'll be able to double my winnings on the one-three-four. Just don't you go and play your mama's little boy game and spill the beans." Martin rocked back and forth on his feet, his clenched boxer's fists jammed into the pockets of his sports jacket. "Look at those damn lines. They're too long. It's only a few minutes till post time. You stay here and I'll move to that shorter line over there. It'll save us some money if you don't get to bet, anyway. How I'm ever gonna turn the business over to you is beyond me," he muttered as he walked away.

"Yeah, okay, Dad, I'll meet you back at the seats."

Both his parents were waiting for him when he got back to the row of seats. The two places on either side of his mother were saved, one for him, one for his father. Naomi loved to sit between them, saying it made her proud for everybody to see what handsome men she lived with.

Joshua always thought they made a strange trio, especially considering the differences in his and Martin's physical appearance. In contrast, Joshua favored Naomi's side of the family.

Martin had always considered his wife's people to be a weak-headed lot, eternally dependent on the whims of fate and a stern, distant God with Whom he himself had ceased to communicate. Martin Caliban's fate was in Martin Caliban's hands. And no other's.

One of the several teams Martin had bet on won. He turned toward his son and opened his clenched fists, revealing a dozen jai alai tickets. Martin ripped the losing tickets to shreds and threw them in the air like confetti.

"I just knew the five and six were sleepers!" he gloated. "I just knew it! At least *someone* in this family knows how to pick a winner."

Joshua's limbs felt heavier and heavier. The dream was beginning to lose its grip and he was sinking deeper into sleep. Ironically, good dreams always ended with his father winning. If Martin lost and Joshua had won, there would have been hell to pay when they got home. Martin would grab his cat-o'-nine-tails before he got halfway into the house, using it on Joshua just to assuage his anger. To Martin Caliban, losing face was worse than losing money—especially to his own son.

Three

Joshua held the prescription bottle up to the light and twisted it
slowly. He liked to watch the capsules shift and slide among
each other through the amber-colored plastic, like the beautiful
shapes of a kaleidoscope. But now there was nothing to see
except the shadows of his fingers. How could he have been so
careless? Had he been dipping into his stash more often lately?

He set the bottle down and flicked on his computer. With
shaking fingers, he stroked the keys that would open to view
C.C.A.'s current pharmacy inventory. "Incorrect code. Access
denied." He must have typed in the wrong code in his haste.

"Slow down, slow down, no need to panic," he whispered.

Not that he couldn't make it through the day without a pill.
He'd done it many times in the past just to prove that he still had
the situation under control. But he couldn't get over his fear that
one day when he really *needed* it, he wouldn't be able to get any.

Joshua took a deep breath and retyped the access code. This
time the pharmacy's logo leaped to the screen. He navigated to
"Controlled Narcotics" and was delighted to see that a new
shipment had just been received. Among the thousands of pre-
scriptions C.C.A. regularly filled, no one would notice the ones
he tapped as long as he didn't stay hooked on any one crutch.
His financial advisors called it "spreading the risk" when
referring to his investment portfolio. The medications he took

31

provided the same kind of insurance, namely keeping him balanced. It was nothing more than a harmless way of investing in his health and well-being, and therefore the health and well-being of C.C.A.

God bless Damien for forcing this lovely system on us, Joshua thought. The computer network that Damien had designed and implemented was so sophisticated that it put C.C.A. on the leading edge of technology. Accessing and controlling information such as this inventory was a snap compared to what it had once been. Thank God Damien had been so vehement about it. The computer system made accessing the drugs possible.

And Damien was nothing if not a control freak. After getting the go-ahead from the board to initiate the expensive computer program, Damien immediately had set up a random drug testing system to guard against the human error he so despised.

Mistakes could be made in entering the correct inventory of pharmaceutical shipments in many ways. Sometimes the drug manufacturers themselves simply mislabeled the quantities of products they delivered. Sometimes one of the pharmacists might accidentally drop a box on the floor. When this happened, the box had to be discounted, because C.C.A.'s policy stated that anything that hit the floor had to be destroyed. Damien referred to people who made these mistakes as "culprits." They were immediately required to complete a special Drug Destruction form—Damien called the D.D.'s his "watchdog." Damien would personally review these forms and God help the employee who had filled it out incorrectly.

"We can't have people in this business who don't follow orders," Damien told Joshua when questioned about his harsh handling of honest mistakes. "Measure me by the results I get with my people, Joshua, not by my methods. When your colleagues don't follow procedures, it costs us millions in malpractice suits. I'm only trying to control costs from my end."

These forms were sent to what the staff referred to as "Command Control," otherwise known as Damien's office. Once there, only a person who knew the secret access code could then effect a change in the inventory by manipulating the numbers on the screen. Naturally, it was Damien, and Damien alone, who possessed the code numbers.

Periodically, Damien would run a spot check of the inventories without announcing it beforehand. One day, while he was implementing one of these watchdog procedures, Joshua wandered into his office unannounced.

Damien had a sinister smile. His beady brown eyes reminded Joshua of a shark's eyes as it circles its prey, anticipating the taste of blood. "Have a seat and I'll be right with you. I'm just cleaning up a discrepancy in the inventory."

Joshua took this as an opportunity presented to him by divine providence if such a thing existed. He zoomed in on Damien's keyboard and screen. Within a few seconds, he'd recorded and memorized both the access procedure and the codes as accurately as if he'd taken a photograph of them.

He could then sneak into the inventory system and adjust the amounts in the computer records whenever he wanted. He always made his visits to the pharmacy to pick up the drugs during the evening hours or on weekends when only a skeleton staff was working. He used the pretext that he was simply stopping by to say hello. This impressed the staff, to see the CEO making the rounds just like a regular guy. Swiping a handful of pills while they were busy working was easy. The few times anyone had taken notice, he'd simply asked for a prescription pad and written a scrip for a small dosage. Two minutes later, he'd be at his computer, correcting the inventory.

His phone buzzed insistently.

"It's ten o'clock, Dr. Caliban, and Dr. King is here to see you," Mary said.

Joshua winced. He had forgotten. He had only agreed to see this woman because of Jane's odd insistence. All he expected to get out of this meeting was to end up even further behind in his work. Damien had been on him for days to catch up on the pile of overdue chart entries, arguing that no one else would follow C.C.A.'s medical records policies if the CEO didn't.

Scrunching the phone between his shoulder and ear, Joshua tried to tidy the paper mess with one hand. The other reached into his bottom desk drawer and searched frantically. Maybe one of his "babies" had fallen into a corner. No luck.

He tried to keep the edge out of his voice: "Is it time already? All right, bring her in, Mary."

Joshua stood abruptly and stretched, nearly knocking askew the magnificent trophy trout frozen in a leap to freedom above his desk.

His stethoscope hung like a talisman around the trout's neck, but Joshua didn't want to put it on. At the moment, it looked too much like a noose. He reached instead for his white coat, which decorated the trout's tail.

The coat was several sizes too big, even for his large frame. As he slid his arms into the sleeves, he felt like Moses assuming his mantle. Well, at least that was what Ruth always told him when he was fully dressed in his medical whites. He knew he presented an imposing figure. The brilliant white of the starched cloth set off his steel-gray hair and beard magnificently, and he'd lost none of the muscle padding in his chest and shoulders that helped fill out the garment's shape. He hoped Dr. King would be suitably impressed—and hopefully, she'd be on her way by the end of the day.

Joshua turned off his computer and glanced at the door to his office. He blinked. Then again. Once more. The bright lights in the hallway backlit the woman's slender, six-foot body and accentuated her long, wavy blonde hair with a silvery glow. She stood perfectly still, smiling. Even with the light in his eyes, the whiteness of her teeth seemed shockingly fluorescent against the cocoa brown color of her skin. It made her smile glow like a jack-o'-lantern. But she certainly did not resemble a pumpkin in any way!

Joshua felt his heart racing. Her beauty was overwhelming. Erect but not rigid, her stance radiated a majesty that the simplicity of her professionally impeccable Armani suit only served to enhance. But the curves clearly and gently swelled under that fine-woven, taupe-colored wool. The images he associated with her played a tug of war in his mind. She was an exotic Nubian queen, supreme in her self-assurance. He was dazed by her slightly almond-shaped eyes. Something in their amber glow echoed the light in his favorite painting, the enigmatic Mona Lisa. Make that the enigmatic and slightly humorous Mona Lisa. He simply *had* to smile back at her.

When she moved toward him she did so effortlessly, extending her hand as she spoke. "Please, stop fussing with your papers. A messy desk is the sign of a creative person. And please don't feel that you have to dress in full uniform," she said still smiling. "My name is Moerae King. It's pronounced like the song, 'they call the wind Mariah.' I'd like it if you called me Moerae. It's a pleasure to meet you."

Not used to feeling like an awkward fourteen year-old, Joshua thrust his hand out over the desk. "I'm Joshua Caliban. Sorry for the mess, anyway, though you're gracious to excuse it. Performing surgery is the least complicated part of this business nowadays. The paperwork really overwhelms me." Her hand was slender and cool to the touch, but the brief pressure she gave him as they released their handshake sent an unexpectedly electric pulse up his arm. "Please, have a seat," he said, pointing to the couch behind the coffee table.

35

Joshua's mind was racing as fast as his pulse as he watched Moerae glide gracefully to a landing in the chair. "It's getting harder and harder to be a good doctor these days," he blurted. Did he sound as foolish to her as he did to himself? He suddenly wished he'd splashed some cologne on his face. A long time had passed since he'd been aroused by any woman other than Ruth.

"The house of Hippocrates seems to be under attack," she said cheerfully. "I hope I can be of some help."

"Well ... yes." He turned away from her eyes, which seemed to see him no matter where he looked. Dammit! If she just weren't so attractive! "Our attorney, Jane Sherwood, heard you speak at the A.B.A. luncheon the other day." He paused in an effort to regain his command of the situation, failed, then continued anyway. "*She* seems to think you can be of some help to us. Can I get you some coffee?"

"Yes, thank you," Moerae said. She shifted slightly as she comfortably crossed her long legs.

"How do you take it?"

"Black is beautiful. Thank you." She winked and flashed that radiant smile again. "And that's a real beauty, too," Moerae said, nodding at the trophy trout. "A fish of that size must have a story attached to it. Is that you in the photograph?"

Joshua looked at the picture of him proudly holding the beautiful trophy, with his father standing alongside mocking the size of the fish with his own hands. He handed Moerae her cup and poured himself one. The last thing he wanted to talk about in this first meeting was the devastating effect his father had had on his life. The seconds of silence expanded until they filled the office, but he noticed that Moerae still hadn't lost the pleasantly expectant expression surrounding her face when she first appeared at his door. "Yes. A somewhat younger model."

"It's truly beautiful. How do they ever get it to look so real?"

Joshua started to relax. Whatever else she might be, Dr. Moerae King wasn't insensitive.

"Do you really want to know? My father, Martin, taught me most of what I know about taxidermy, and it pretty much comes down to one simple rule. In the first place, you have to know that you want to keep the fish before you kill it because *how* you kill it is the trick. You have to do it humanely. If something has to die, you do it swiftly, cleanly and carefully. You don't torture it or allow it to suffer."

"That's why I never enjoyed fishing," Moerae said. "I can't bear to kill anything. But what does it mean to *carefully* kill something?"

"Usually, if I'm planning just to take the fish home to grill, I use a small wooden club to bang it over the bridge of its nose. But my father taught me that you never do that to a trophy fish because it mars the skin."

She tilted her blond head, the light dazzling upon it, and massaged her left palm with her right thumb. "So, how do you handle a fish like that one if you want it to be a trophy?"

Joshua shivered. "You have to drive a sharp, pointed object into the eyeball forcefully enough to pierce the fish's brain."

Moerae swallowed the last of her coffee and put down the cup on the table. "Thank you, that was lovely. But I've distracted you into telling me fishing stories. Let's get down to business, shall we? It sounded like your attorney thought I could help, but you're not too sure." Her voice rose with a slight question-mark tone.

"Well frankly, Dr. King, like most health care organizations, our greatest threats come in the form of attacks from several different quarters: from the sharks—er, sorry, lawyers—to those bloodsuckers in Washington who think they've been elected to reform the health system in this country. I find it hard to see how organizational psychology can offer much help. And to be truthful, I'm not even sure I know what it is."

Moerae uncrossed her legs and leaned forward, a slight wrinkle crossed her brow. "Yes, Dr. Caliban, you're certainly not alone in the challenges you face. Nor is the field of health care unique in its sense of being under attack. In fact, I can't think of a single institution in this country that isn't suffering from growing pains. Families, schools, small businesses, government agencies, even those sharks and Washington leeches you refer to—they all need help."

Joshua waved his finger in front of his face, brushing the tip of his nose. "There's one thing Jane mentioned that intrigues me. She said you made the comment that organizations act just like individual people. I think I know what you mean, but I wouldn't be able to give you a definition. The theory sounds interesting, but I don't see how treating an organization as a person will help me be a better CEO."

Moerae nodded and leaned back. "Fair enough. Let me try to give you a practical explanation." She looked again at the fish on the wall. "You're a trout fisherman and, obviously, a very accomplished one at that. A man couldn't bag such a magnificent, wild creature as that without possessing great singularity of purpose and commitment. It's a real achievement."

Joshua grinned and his cheeks felt flush. Moerae King was a good listener. And despite the fact that she was clearly an intelligent and skillful player, he also felt sure that her appreciation was genuine, which warmed him to her even more than her physical beauty.

"Now, let me ask you this: How many of the leaders—let alone the rank and file staff workers—share your drive and commitment to the vision and mission of C.C.A.?"

The question found the bull's eye of its intended target. Joshua suddenly felt very alone with his dream of what C.C.A. could yet become. Sure, sometimes a few of his colleagues showed commitment to excellence more than to the bottom line. . . but did anyone really understand his vision—that steely determination forged in the heated frustration that tore at him during his Cook County residency? The look on his face answered her query.

"Bear with me, now," she said, "I sometimes sound like I'm up on a soapbox once I get going."

Joshua waved a hand. "No, go ahead. It's actually refreshing to hear someone speak with a little passion and commitment."

She took a deep breath, and the fire in her eyes revealed just a hint of her ardor. "I believe that our fundamental problem—that which is eating the foundations out from under our crumbling institutions—is a kind of *spiritual bankruptcy*." She let the words sink in, then leaned forward and held up her manicured fingers to count. "Let me give you a couple of examples:

"First, the easy targets: scandal-ridden politics. Doesn't it seem the last half of the twentieth century was just one huge downward slide for American governmental institutions? Does anyone believe or respect government leaders or agencies anymore? Self-centered politicos, drunk with power and their own self-importance deliver crushing blows to American political idealism every day as they enact legislation creating unfair advantage—and even monopolies— for self-serving special interest groups. And the personal scandals in the lives of national leaders only demonstrate how morally rudderless we've become.

"Then look to Wall Street. The heady days of the 1990s saw unimaginable amounts of cash flowing into the markets. It was fueled by the insatiable greed of get-rich-quick American investors—it was like visiting the casinos of Vegas. And the recipients of all this wealth—the heads of new, fast-growing corporations—found themselves riding a wave of cash and power that gripped them with an addiction as potentially lethal as any mind-altering substance or toxic drug you could ingest or inject!"

Joshua twitched and glanced quickly at the drawer under his desk, but Moerae didn't seem to notice.

"Senior executives rewarded themselves with *un–be–liev–a–ble* salaries and benefits! All the while, their corporations returned little value for the investments made by hard-working investors. CEOs and their cronies act as though their subordinates are too stupid to notice that they themselves don't follow the very policies and procedures they enact. They dehumanize and objectify their workers. They've lost sight—and not only they but many of us, individually and collectively, have lost sight of our fundamental reason for being."

"So are you saying what we need is some old-time religion?" Joshua sarcastically exaggerated his incredulity.

"Hardly! Most organized religions have simply tried to dictate morality to us using tired, cliché-filled sermons—little more than rehearsed rhetoric delivered from the pulpit by a clergyman who seems completely out of touch. Few church-goers ever hear anything delivered from the heart—an original or exciting thought. How can they find a real purpose for their existence there? And to finish off any remaining credibility, congregants are sick of religious hierarchies infected with the same addiction to power contaminating Wall Street and the government!"

"The deepening spiritual bankruptcy of our society's leaders trickles down—no, *cascades* down throughout our culture. The heads of our families follow the lead of our heads of state. How else can you explain the reported cases of child abuse that exceed four million this year alone?"

Taken aback by the fervor of her "sermon," Joshua grunted and cleared his throat. He signaled his reservations by stroking the skin under his bearded chin. "You'd make a good judge,

Dr. King. Did you ever study law? You sum it up very succinctly. You won't be getting any argument from my side. Believe me, I've become all too familiar with many kinds of abuse in my practice and in my life. The world is most assuredly in a sorry state of affairs, but I still fail to see what the number of child abuse cases has to do with whatever is troubling health care in general—or C.C.A. in particular. We treat these casualties every day, Dr. King. We don't cause them."

Moerae lowered her chin and glanced down at the floor. "I apologize," she said in a more subdued tone. "I warned you, I tend to get on my high horse occasionally. Perhaps I could show a connection between all of this and your bottom line if I knew a little more about you and where you stand on a few issues. May I ask you a few questions?"

"Please do."

Moerae paused and cupped her chin in her hand. "Have you ever observed one of your colleagues chewing out some nurse's ass?"

Joshua raised an eyebrow in surprised amusement. A moment before, she'd sounded almost like a professor of philosophy expounding on the state of the world. But now she had succeeded in drawing his full attention. Judging from the mischievous smile playing on her full mouth, that had been her intention.

Joshua chuckled and nodded. "I'm sure I've done it more than once myself. But that's to be expected in a high-pressure business like ours. We deal constantly in matters of life and death. And in the heat of daily battle, sometimes we lose sight of the fact that our workers are human, too. But what does that have to do with our ailing bottom line?"

Moerae returned his chuckle. "It's the shrink in me. They taught us basic skills like how to talk in circles in Psych 101. But let me be direct: Treating subordinate workers disrespectfully injures more than the person who is belittled. It injures your organization. And we can't simply wash away the pain and suffering caused by our behavior toward each other by issuing a half-hearted apology later on.

"In your work as a surgeon, you know you can swab the blood off the floor of the O.R. after open-heart surgery and erase all the traces of what has happened in that room. But the heart, even as it's healing, will still carry a memory of what it has experienced as surely as it carries scars in its tissues."

Another shot on target. The Mayos and Kaisers certainly taught her a few things about medicine, Joshua thought as he stroked his beard and beckoned her to continue.

"Let me give you another medical analogy. You know how a staph infection that's contracted in the operating room can be potentially lethal. It can prohibit the process of healing to the point of causing death. What I propose is that a *staff* infection— S-T-A-F-F—is an equally toxic, unhealthy relationship between two or more human beings anywhere within the corporation. And it can be just as deadly for the whole organization. It stunts growth, cripples functionality and can eventually kill it. That's because a company or any business is every bit as organic as a human being. Being made up of humans, it's just as complex, just as alive, and just as full of potential for life … or death. And it's true whether you're talking about a school caring for young minds, a church ministering to lost souls, or a hospital working to repair broken bones and ailing hearts."

"I don't know about all this touchy-feely stuff …" Joshua began.

Moerae interrupted, "At the risk of being out of line, I'd like to point out that in your business touchy-feely shouldn't be considered a negative. After all, people get in touch with you when they need to feel better."

Moerae flashed him the jack-o'-lantern teeth, disarming the growing uneasiness in his gut. He wasn't used to feeling backed into an intellectual corner. In his childhood, he'd played word games with his mother, and those pleasurable, quiet afternoons exercising his mind in her gentle company had led him to pursue words well into his adult life. He seldom lost a verbal sparring match with anyone.

"Yes, Ms. Sherwood told me about your theory correlating the behavior of those in the boardroom to their behavior in the operating room. And I can *certainly* hear and respect your commitment to the health care profession."

"I do apologize if I sounded like I was singling out the health care industry," Moerae said, not sounding apologetic at all. Quite the opposite, as a matter of fact: She seemed totally self-possessed. But she didn't sound as though she were being sarcastic either.

Staring evenly at him, her amber eyes unblinking, she said, "I have absolutely no doubt that you feel as deeply as I do that human beings in need of repair deserve a better deal than their cars might get."

His skin prickled. Car dealerships. A small rush of adrenaline surged through him. Had she actually researched his own history so far as to discover his father's livelihood? So what else did she already know about him? He felt exposed. This woman had either done her homework or could catch a trout like his by casting blind.

Clearing his throat again, he asked, "Do you have experience in the automotive industry as well? Perhaps that would help me to get a better handle on how, if at all, *you* might be able to help *me*."

Moerae deliberately picked up her briefcase and laid it on her lap. The snap of the locks as she released them made a quietly authoritative sound. She leafed briefly through an envelope, then passed the newspaper clipping she pulled out to Joshua. "No, but I did have an opportunity to work with the airline industry. You might recall this article in the *Times* about TransCentral Airlines a few years back."

Joshua blinked at the headline in heavy black ink that stood out boldly on the page. He pulled his reading glasses from his pocket. A flood of painful memories flashed across his mind He remembered this headline very well. Ruth's parents had died on a TransCentral flight. At the time, he'd read no further than the words he saw in front of him now: *Hatred Poisoned and Killed TransCentral Airlines.*

"The combatants dug in more deeply and actually began to look forward to a strike so they finally could tear at each other's throats ... the hate won't dissipate ... the poison is still so strong that some machinists cheered last week when TransCentral went dark with not a trace of concern for the customers who have lost a major carrier, or for the fact that they themselves had lost employment."

Moerae began slowly. "What's not mentioned in that editorial are the results of the F.A.A. safety report done on the accident. Its conclusion stated that the extent of the anger and hatred ravaging the organization had grown so great, it was like a cancer, which I quote, 'could easily impact the safety of the millions of passengers who put their lives into TransCentral's hands every day.'"

Joshua laughed nervously. "I can see why the media would want to suppress that choice little bit of information. If the sharks had gotten hold of that, they would've gone into a full feeding frenzy!"

Moerae continued in a soft, measured voice that had a near hypnotic effect on Joshua. "Where does venom like that come from? Such suicidal behavior, as the editorial labeled it? It has to start with the policies, the personal behaviors and procedures

---

dictated by whoever is in the boardroom. And even if their dictates were benign originally, aren't those leaders still accountable?"

The intercom buzzed as if in a distant dream, over and over. Finally startled, he leaned over and pushed the intercom button.

"Your reservations at La Boheme are for twelve-thirty, Dr. Caliban."

"Thank you, Mary."

He sighed with relief and shook off the spell. "I took the liberty of making us reservations at one of those nouvelle cuisine places. You know the ones, small dishes with big prices. I can cancel it if that doesn't suit you."

"That would be lovely," she said smiling. She stood and floated gracefully toward the office door. "Just give me a moment to powder my nose and I'll be ready to go."

"Feel free to use mine," he offered, pointing to the private bathroom at the rear of his office. "We still have a few executive perks."

Joshua couldn't help staring at her as she passed. Her flowing, richly blonde hair captured even the pale glow of the office overhead lights and reflected back a subdued yet vibrant glow. She seemed a study in contrasts and yet she was clearly self-possessed—whole.

Was her hair naturally blonde? Would he ever know?

Four

Animated conversations sparkled around the room at La Boheme, enhanced by martinis and wine. This restaurant was a meeting place for all the power brokers of Chicago. Everyone present for lunch had an agenda. The patterns of speech, subtle body movements and deliberate pauses in conversation made clear to even a casual observer how the pecking order was arranged at each of the small tables.

Joshua and Moerae followed the maitre d' to the window table that Joshua always reserved. Their progress seemed to carve a swath of silence through the room as all chatter and animation suspended breathlessly as they passed each table. Mocrae nodded and smiled politely as Joshua acknowledged Andrew Polanski, the city commissioner of insurance, who waved discreetly from his table.

Joshua lowered his head and whispered, "He's a contemporary sort of Robin Hood, only reversed. He steals from the poor to line the pockets of the rich."

Virgil Carter sat with Andrew. Joshua mirrored Andrew's weak smile with one of his own. "One of the sharks! We've butted heads several times," he whispered through gritted teeth.

"I'll bet his still hurts," Moerae whispered back.

Joshua knew that Carter would be bursting to update his crony—and chair of the Young Presidents Club, Shelly Jackson, what he had witnessed at lunch: Joshua Caliban was dining with a smashing-looking mulatto giantess, replete with startling amber eyes set like jewels in a face carved of mahogany.

Once they were seated and had ordered, Joshua interrogated Moerae as if taking her personal history and physical. Her father had been an Afro-American merchant seaman from Chicago and her mother, Greek. They'd met in Athens, fallen in love tumultuously and emphatically, married and moved to the United States within a month's time. Moerae seemed proud that her passionate parents had been practical enough to have known what they wanted in a mate and to also have had the sense to recognize it in each other almost instantaneously—despite their different backgrounds.

Tragically, both had been killed in an automobile accident when she was a teenager. Moerae was raised by her father's middle-class family until she graduated from high school. It was from her grandmother that she'd acquired her love of books and her consuming interest in studying human nature. The older woman was something of a self-taught savant and was recognized by her neighbors as being a natural healer and wise woman.

Moerae grew up uniquely poised between two cultures—her grandparents taught her to be proud of her dual heritage. From early on she determined to be mistress of her own destiny. Moerae King would never depend on anyone else to earn her keep. She put herself through the University of Chicago doing any kind of work that would fit her class schedule—from waiting tables in greasy spoons to delivering room service to businessmen in the best hotels in the city. Joshua couldn't help smiling when she wryly remarked how these experiences taught her more about human behavior than the best of her psych courses.

Moerae had also inherited a passion for philosophy from her mother and had been particularly attracted to Zen Buddhism. When she described her favorite exercise for developing concentration, which was watching her breath move in and out through the tip of her nose, he remarked that it reminded him of the qualities a good trout fisherman needed.

"You see," she said, "we have more in common than you thought. I'm not a fisherman, but I'll bet we share many other qualities, too."

"All right, what about sports. Are you a Cubs fan?"

Moerae's amber eyes opened exaggeratedly wide and her slender hands pointed innocently back at herself. A teasing smile crossed her full lips. "Oh, no!" she exclaimed. "I would never abuse myself so much. I don't foster hopes and dreams that can't be fulfilled."

"Are you telling me you're one of those damned Yankees?"

"To the core."

"Well, I won't count that against you. By the way, I'm very curious about your name. It's quite unusual."

She nodded. "That's what people say. My father wanted to name me Jemima, after his mother. But my mother was dead set against it. No daughter of hers was going to be named after a pancake mix. It didn't take her long, you understand, to become acculturated in this country. That's an innate talent the Greeks have."

"Yet your mother sounds like she had a mind of her own." Joshua paused and let his narrowed eyes fix softly on Moerae's. "After all, she came halfway around the world to be with your father and start a new life in a foreign country. Yes, I'd say she'd have been a very strong character. Rather like you. You must take after her."

Moerae smiled and nodded, her eyes suddenly bright with tears. She quickly blinked a few times, took a deep breath, and let it out slowly through her pursed lips. "She had a theory about names, but I won't bore you with it now."

Joshua leaned forward and placed his hand briefly on hers, then put it back on the table. "Please, I want to hear it. We're in no rush. I sometimes wonder if *nouvelle cuisine* is a French term for 'very slow service.' We might not eat for hours."

Moerae leaned forward, put her elbow on the table and rested her chin in the palm of her hand. "My mother came from a very religious Greek Orthodox family. In addition to the traditional beliefs she learned from her parents, she had a special reverence for what she called the sacred order underlying the things of this world. Her spiritual nature was so honest and simple, it had to rub off on anyone who spent time with her. She taught me what she believed, that we choose our own parents before birth. We choose them for their strengths *and* weaknesses so that the proper opportunities will present themselves in our lives to play out our karmic scripts."

"A very solemn viewpoint, indeed, and contrary to the common notion of destiny, if I get your drift. It puts the responsibility for our lives back on each one of us. And if it's true," he said, laughing ruefully, "I made a very poor choice for myself."

Moerae raised her neatly penciled cocoa-brown eyebrows. When Joshua didn't elaborate, she continued, "First names, on the other hand, are given. Parents often imprint their children with first names that carry the weight of their own unrealized hopes, fears or dreams—all unconsciously, of course."

Moerae sipped her water, watching as Joshua reached for his water glass at the same instant. "So, hypothetically speaking, a Joshua's life would be likely to fight more battles—battles of Jericho?—than, say, a man named John Doe." She smiled warmly at him.

"And … ?" Joshua asked, smiling back.

"Me?" Her smooth skin wrinkled around her almond eyes as she scrunched up her face girlishly. "My mother told me my eyes reminded her of Moerae, the Greek goddess of destiny. She said their color made them look bottomless, like a seer's eyes, looking into a deep spring of clear water. I guess it came from a habit I had from when I was a small child, of staring out the window, daydreaming. She always told me I'd grow up to be an advisor to kings, or, at the very least, a counselor to great men." Moerae laughed, shrugged her shoulders and held her hands out, palms up. "Looks like she was right!"

Not until they'd finished their meal and were having their coffee did he finally get around to saying, in a slightly halting way, "I see that you're wearing a wedding ring. I must have misunderstood Ms. Sherwood. She gave me the impression that you were unattached. What does your husband do for a living?"

Moerae shifted backwards, rubbed her thumb into the palm of her hand, and gazed down at her ring. After a moments silence, she leaned forward. "I noticed you staring at my ring—no, don't bother to apologize. It's only natural that you'd be curious. And I'll admit that I've pondered how I'll answer you. Because I want all of our dealings with each other to be open, I'll tell you the truth. My significant other is one of those sharks you so dislike." She paused long enough for Joshua to catch her eyes sparkling. "She's a lawyer."

Joshua's broad shoulders snapped to attention. He blurted, "Oh, I didn't mean to pry. I'm sorry I asked." Heat rose in his cheeks. "I have a confession, too. I'll admit to you freely that, in spite of the fact that I'm very much in love with my wife, your sheer beauty has given rise to some harmless fantasies about you. Now that you've dashed cold water on them, I'll have to replace them with some new ones." He flashed her one of his most artless grins.

"Well, your candor utterly charms me, Dr. Caliban," she said in an exaggerated southern drawl. "But seriously, I'm very glad that you asked. I knew you'd wonder and I wouldn't have felt comfortable not being honest with you. My partner and I are deeply in love, physically and emotionally, but the best part of our being together is that we often find ourselves on the same side of serious issues. Otherwise, I doubt we would have lasted this long. I can be pretty intense sometimes, especially where my work is concerned."

Joshua's shoulders relaxed and he nodded several times. "Then we have still another thing in common. My wife says the same thing about me."

"But the best part is that both my partner and I believe our relationship to be fundamentally very practical." She laughed, the impish sparkle of her eyes and tilted head inviting him to respond.

He rose to the bait. "Practical? You sure know how to confuse a guy! From everything you've told me so far today, I never would expect you to refer to love and intimacy as 'practical'! Help me understand what you mean."

She held up three fingers triumphantly and, one by one, counted them off. "One, you never have to worry about birth control. Two, there are no scratchy beards to irritate the skin. And, last but not least, the toilet seat is always left down."

Joshua laughed until the tears came to his eyes. Moerae threw her head back and laughed as well.

"You're a rare and engaging person, Moerae, and I must say that I've thoroughly enjoyed our lunch. But it takes more than charm and wit to run a health care organization; I'm a person who deals best in concrete terms, and so are my colleagues on the board. Simply put, how can you help us?"

Moerae smiled radiantly. "First let me say how pleased I am to see our potential for being friends—regardless of whether we go further. If we *do* work together, that will become more and more important as time goes by. Your openness has already given me a much better idea of how to frame my prescription for C.C.A., but I'd like to mull it over in private for a while before sending you a written proposal."

Joshua nodded.

"I won't start the meter running unless you decide to continue with me—*after* you study my proposal to your satisfaction. I promise to make it as concrete and practical as I can," Moerae said. "The next few days are very busy for me, as I have heavy client commitments, but I can have the proposal on your desk in less than two weeks. Will that work for you?"

"It's an offer I can hardly refuse. Are you sure you don't have any experience selling cars, Moerae?"

She stood up, laughing, and pretended to roll up her sleeves. "Joshua, have I got a deal for you! I'll match any offer you or Ruth get from any other dealer in town!"

"How did you know Ruth's … oh, never mind," Joshua said, shaking his head. He'd probably mentioned Ruth's name to Moerae some time during the last couple of hours. "I must be off, now, to save a few bleeding hearts." Joshua assumed a gallant air, rose from his chair, and reached out to take her hand. "Can I drop you off somewhere, or did you drive to the hospital this morning?"

"No, thank you. I've got a few errands to run downtown and, since I'm a shopping addict, I'll take the opportunity to pick up a few things. Then I'll catch a cab back to my office."

They retraced their path through the tables, the other patrons staring. From the doorway, Moerae paused and, turning slightly, took a long, leisurely look at the room over her shoulder. She smiled and turning back to the door Joshua held open for her, walked regally out.

❦

Damien Rees stole a careful look from a corner table wedged deliberately behind one of the imported Italian marble columns. He breathed a sigh of relief that he'd managed to remain undetected by Joshua for the entire meal. He didn't want to run into him just yet. There didn't seem to be much danger of that, judging from the absorbed attention Joshua had lavished on his lunch partner. She was a looker all right—even though she wasn't Damien's type.

Yes, he was very pleased he'd been able to observe without being seen especially in light of recent events. That closed meeting behind his back, for example. As the only regular board member who hadn't attended, he was pretty sure the subject matter must have been him. Big deal. He had his ways of finding out what had been on the agenda.

He was similarly pleased that he hadn't had to make kissy-face with Joshua in the middle of a discussion over steak tartar with Ashton Simons. Ashton, president of Big Blue, the largest third-party payer in town, had the unwitting grace to disappear into the men's room shortly before Joshua and that amazing woman had made their grand entrance. Blond haired mulatto. Must be some story there.

Joshua's back had been to them all during lunch. Although connecting regularly with Ashton was routine for him, Damien nevertheless disliked mixing his business. And—more importantly—he didn't want to give C.C.A.'s CEO any reason to wonder about his relationship with Ashton. What the left hand didn't know about the right hand's activities was all to the good.

In fact, Damien and Ashton had been doing business through a special arrangement for several years. Ashton had initially contacted him after seeing the results of Damien's billing system. Ashton was convinced that it was Damien's own computer wizardry that streamlined the process and minimized the time between a patient's visit and billing for its appropriate insurance payment. He just couldn't get over it.

"I've never seen anyone get their doctors to sign a patient's billing papers so fast. What's the incentive? Do you stand over them with a stick? I didn't think there'd be a carrot big enough to get their attention. Those guys already have more money than God."

"Oh, it was easy," Damien told him, flattered in spite of himself. "All I had to do was point out to them that the longer we took to bill, the more money you guys made."

"You're a man after my own heart, Damien," Ashton had said, chuckling, his fat stomach jiggling. Damien chuckled, too, but he cringed inwardly as Ashton clapped him heartily on the back.

Ashton and Damien had worked out a simple scheme that served them both well. On the fifteenth of every month, Big Blue made an estimated payment to C.C.A. based on projected billings. This assured C.C.A. of a constant stream of cash without delays. The difference between the actual and estimated billings would be made up at year's end in the final accounting. The challenge was finding how to invest these reserves prudently and to the benefit of Big Blue's many health care providers.

Ashton and Damien were so successful that Ashton formally invited Damien to join Big Blue's board of directors. Joshua's response to this was, "Join their board of directors? Splendid! Having one of ours as a representative in that den of thieves, and at their request, is a wonderful idea! Our board will love it, too."

And as icing on the cake, Damien raked in an additional twenty-thousand a year from his position on Big Blue's board. For once, the physicians at C.C.A. didn't say boo, and anyway, C.C.A.'s employment policy about discretionary income for non-physicians was vague.

For Damien, the money was doubly sweet: Nothing gave him more pleasure than playing both ends against the middle—and winning.

On the other hand, Damien had hidden dues to pay. If not for their special arrangement, Damien wouldn't be caught dead with a man like Ashton Simons. His advanced obesity made his body appear to be nearly spherical. How thoroughly undisciplined the man was. If Ashton couldn't control his own behavior, how could he hope to control anyone else's?

As if to highlight his disgust, Ashton was at that very moment stuffing an entire bread roll into his gaping mouth. Hopefully, it would at least dislodge the piece of spinach in between his bucked front teeth.

"Did you see that front page press Blue Cross of Michigan just got?" Ashton said between bites. He shifted a wad of bread to the opposite cheek and gulped a mouthful of Mouton Cadet to wash it down. "Every health care organization in the country is staggering under a load of financial pressure. More and more of those guys are asking their banks to extend and increase their lines of credit. It's getting very dicey out there. For instance, look at what happened to your competitor, Mackinaw HealthCare. Sure, it's one of those smaller outfits. But I understand their bank foreclosed on their loan just last week." Ashton sucked on his tooth thoughtfully.

"Yes, I heard about that," Damien snapped. God, the big slob made him homicidal! Would he ever get to the point?

"Relax, Damien, don't get your balls all in an uproar. I can see you're getting nervous with me," Ashton said, leaning forward. "Well, the banks are caught in a damned-if-you-do, damned-if-you-don't type of situation. The bank certainly wanted to get its money out, but it's a sure thing that if they force an organization to shut its doors, they're never going to see a penny. So Blue Cross comes up with this strategy. They figure a lot of patients are going to lose their health care, too, and that's important to them. So it makes a lot of sense for them to hire somebody to try to turn the situation around. And guess what?" Ashton sat back, beaming. "What better choice than good old Big Blue? We understand the business as well, if not better, than anyone else."

"Ashton, I'm telling you, I read the article. Don't talk to me like I'm some rookie M.B.A. student," Damien said, gritting his teeth behind his curled lips. "We were talking about the relative pros and cons of changing C.C.A.'s baseline monthly reimbursement figure. Let me reiterate our reasoning. C.C.A.'s billings have been showing noticeable signs of growth. That means expenses are increasing. C.C.A. is going to need more frequent increments of operating capital, so if Big Blue's monthly reimbursements don't increase accordingly, C.C.A. is going to be forced to ask for a bigger line of credit with its own bank. We know it'll all wash out when the final, end-of-year adjustments are made in December. Are you with me so far?"

"Sure, sure, Damien. Go ahead and spell it out."

Damien sighed and then took a deep breath. The man has a mind like Swiss cheese. "On the other hand, we agree that if the recent increase proves to be just a flash in the pan, it doesn't make good business sense to increase the baseline payments prematurely. If we do that, we run the risk of having to make another adjustment downward."

"These are hard times," Ashton said with a huff. "If management were prudent, it would hold the line for at least another year. That way, we can see if the increase in actual billings is short-term, or is, in fact, indicative of an overall increase in business. What do you think?"

"If a case like that came before me as a CEO, I think I'd be inclined to take the conservative position, too. I'd rather be the bearer of unexpectedly good news in December than try to ride out a roller coaster during the whole year. People get upset by constant up-and-down changes. They like the straight and narrow, it makes them feel secure." Damien reached for the check that had just arrived.

Ashton reached for the check at the same time, but his stuttering movement showed that his heart wasn't in it. "May I? You paid the last time," Ashton said.

"You can owe me one," Damien said. He enjoyed keeping people indebted to him, and Ashton might be particularly useful one day. If C.C.A. should ever fire him, Ashton would be the one to provide him safe passage through hostile territory into the waiting arms of Big Blue.

Damien fantasized how, as executive vice president, he could put the squeeze on C.C.A.'s cash flow and throw the bank into full panic. Just like Blue Cross, who could better take over running the badly bleeding Care Corporation of America than Big Blue? And how deliciously ironic that he, the ex-chief operating officer of C.C.A., would then be in full control of his former employer.

Ashton pushed his massive bulk away from the table with difficulty. He spoke only half in jest. "I'm sure you won't forget to keep track of the interest."

❧

Joshua dashed into the O.R., gently pinching Kathy Marshall's rounded posterior as she bent over the sterilizer. Kathy had been his head nurse for years. An attractive brunette who combined compassion, skill, and toughness, she had won Joshua's respect over the many years they'd worked together.

"Hey, watch it, watch it," she said sternly. "You wanna get slapped with a harassment suit?"

"How long have I known you, Kath?" Joshua said in feigned innocence. "I just wanted to get your attention. You know I'd never dream of harassing you." He winked. "I meant it in a purely avuncular way." They smiled at each other.

"Yeah," she said, "avuncular, my foot. You're not old enough to be my uncle, so how do you expect anyone to swallow that line?"

"We nipped that rumor in the bud ages ago."

"You mean the one about how we were lovers from the first week we started working together?" Kathy laughed.

"Yeah, that one. I regret it, though. Our discretion. It was kinda fun, wasn't it? Being an item before we'd even shaken hands properly? And, I want to make it perfectly clear, it isn't as though I don't find you attractive."

Kathy shook her head. "Get outta here."

"So, what's the table d'hote this afternoon?"

Without lifting her head, Kathy said, "After what I heard you had for lunch, I'm surprised you have any room left."

"And just how do you know what I had for lunch? It seems I'm the only person in this whole outfit that can't keep a secret. And besides, I was asking him," Joshua shot back, nodding in Peter's direction.

Peter Albert paused in the doorway, clutching his ever-present clipboard with short pudgy fingers. "Nothing special on the menu today," he said. "Pretty standard fare. One double bypass."

Peter Albert hardly looked the part of Joshua's protégé. Joshua's huge, muscular frame often dwarfed Peter's short, chunky one. People called them Mutt and Jeff, although never to Joshua's face. Nevertheless, Peter had a mind as sharp as a scalpel. Placing first in his graduating class, he found it fairly easy to persuade Joshua to offer him the chief residency at C.C.A.

During his first year, Peter's performance had been so out-standing that Joshua had given him a permanent position *pro forma*, in spite of his youth and clumsy looking fingers. The rumor mill went crazy with that one. After all, Peter was young enough to be Joshua's son, and was certainly the youngest doctor ever to be elected to the board of directors. Arguing that C.C.A. needed new blood, Joshua's persistence finally paid off.

In the following months and years with Peter at his side in the operating room, Joshua's appreciation for Peter's other more personal qualities deepened as well. His unfailing loyalty complemented an honesty that could be brutal at times. And most of all, Peter earned Joshua's love with his remarkable ability to deliver the truth with an endearing mixture of tongue-in-cheek humor and earnest seriousness.

Joshua sensed something more, and flexing his fingers in the gloves Kathy fitted over his hands, he queried, "'Pretty standard fare,' you say? I gather there might be some complications in this case. What do we need to watch for?" After hundreds of hours together, Joshua could almost read Peter's mind.

"It's Mrs. Wong," Peter stated.

Ah. Mrs. Wong was almost a celebrity in the hospital. Thanks to Paul Blake's screw up two years ago during her first bypass, she actually died on the operating table. But Joshua managed to bring her back. Then he made a point of greeting her in the recovery room himself, so he could be the first thing she saw when she opened her eyes.

"I'm sorry, madam, but I simply couldn't allow you to take off for Heaven yet. You still have an important place here. We'd miss you too much if you left. Don't you ever try a stunt like that again, do you hear?"

"Thanks, J.C.," she'd whispered groggily. "You don't mind if I call you that, do you? You certainly know how to hold a girl's interest, and naturally, I wouldn't want to leave such a handsome devil as you in the lurch." Her wrinkled face had crinkled up into a smile before she'd slipped back into sleep again.

At seventy-two years old, Susan Wong had known enormous hardship. While she'd been away at boarding school in England, an earthquake in China took her entire family. An Uncle who taught Physics at Northwestern took her in. On top of that, numerous surgeries had badly weakened her body. But nothing ever seemed to dampen her spirits. She had such a good nature, always thinking of someone else. When she was discharged, the staff gave her an "Honorary Mom" plaque. Nevertheless, her family was balking at the prospect of this second bypass. Money wasn't the problem. A sudden windfall of cash they had received would cover the difference between what Medicare and Medicaid would pay. They just didn't want her to suffer anymore.

Joshua looked around the operating room. Everything was ready. He had warned Mrs. Wong of the risks involved with this procedure, but she'd brushed him off. "Everyone's days are numbered you know, dear," she'd said. "Only God knows when my bingo card will fill up. My job is to live as fully as I can until that time comes. So if you're not willing to do the operation, J.C., I'll get another one of God's handymen to do the job."

"That's unfair. You know perfectly well I wouldn't let anyone else touch you."

She was rolled into the room on a gurney with a tube containing a fluid sedative inserted in her left arm. But she was still alert enough to greet everyone in the room as if all were old friends. When she saw Joshua, her narrowing brown eyes lit up and she reached out her free hand to him. "Is my table ready? I made reservations for a window seat. It always does my heart good to see the flowers outside, and that's why we're here, isn't it? To do my heart good."

"Yes and yes. Your table is ready and we are going to do your heart good, Mrs. Wong. It's delightful to see you again."

"You're a marvelous *maitre d'*, J.C. Remind me to leave you a big tip when lunch is over."

Joshua took her hand in his, even though it meant he'd have to re-scrub and re-glove. Through the paper-thin rubber, he could feel the soft skin of her frail, little girl's fingers. So fragile. A lump formed in his throat. He swallowed hard.

"You know the menu, Mrs. Wong. Were there any specials you'd like to hear about before your nap?"

She gazed up into his masked face. "Yes, actually, there is. I'd like to be kissed by a handsome prince before I go to sleep. That way, I know I'll wake up with love in my heart. Promise not to tell Henry though. You know how jealous some men can be even if you've been married to them for over fifty years," she said, her wrinkled grey eyebrows struggling to remain open. "I'll let you do the honors today."

Joshua felt his face flush beneath his mask and was glad no one could read his feelings. "Of course, I'd be honored. But you'll have to grant me a wish, too, fair princess. You must promise never, ever to sue me for sexual harassment." Impulsively, he added, "Plus, you have to return the favor when you wake up."

Susan Wong playfully waggled the finger of her other hand without disturbing her IV. "I must reprimand you. That's two wishes. But since I'm old enough to be your mother, I accept."

Joshua bent to her face and pressed his paper-covered lips tenderly to her cheek.

"It's too bad about that mask," she murmured, fading into unconsciousness. "You'd think I was being kissed by the Lone Ranger rather than a handsome prince."

"Hospital rules, Mrs. Wong. We're required to practice safe sex at all times." Joshua nodded to the anesthesiologist. The short countdown began while Joshua changed his gloves.

For the next hour, the procedure went smoothly, carried along by intermittent conversation.

"So who was that woman you had lunch with? asked Peter, voicing the question on everyone's mind, "Is she a new patient?" Then he added with an audible smirk, "When do we get to massage *her* lungs?"

"Her name is Dr. Moerae King. She's a consultant Jane found for us. I've hired her to help me keep hormonally ravaged, teenage prima donnas like you in line," Joshua answered. "Seriously, Peter, I suspect she might be able to offer us some real help. I'm still learning about what she has to offer, but so far I'm very impressed with what she had to say and how she presented herself. But I don't expect the board will like it, particularly since she doesn't come cheap."

"Sounds to me like you've made up *your* mind," Peter replied.

"Well, I guess maybe I have," Joshua chuckled as he tied a suture. "I surprise even myself." He glanced up over his mask at Peter and rolled his eyes in a full circle. He didn't want the entire hospital to know what he was up to before he told the board. "We'll have to discuss the details later."

Joshua pulled off his gloves. "You can finish sewing up for me, Peter. And please be sure that Mrs. Wong is sent to the new intensive care unit."

Peter raised an eyebrow. The new unit on the other side of the hospital had huge floor-to-ceiling windows looking out onto the garden outside the hospital.

"She does deserve special treatment, doesn't she?" Peter said softly.

"I promised her a rose garden," Joshua replied.

Five

The pulsating jets of water streaming from the shower felt delicious. Finally getting rid of the stale air that circulates on planes, her hair squeaked as she ran and squeezed her hands through it. Ruth's mind played across the long row of pastel silk blouses hanging in her closet. Crushed lapis would go great with the new mohair skirt she'd bought, along with the robin's egg blue on her toenails. Joshua loved the way she color-matched her outfits, and that pleased her immensely. So many of her patients who had suffered sexual abuse as children hated their bodies. Her love for her body was hard-earned and a full wardrobe was her just reward.

The doorbell rang downstairs. Ruth reached for the knob blindly and turned off the water. Stepping from the shower, she grabbed a robe that hung on the back of the door. The smooth, expensive silk whispered over her skin.

"Flowers for Dr. Ruth Caliban," announced the delivery boy standing in her doorway. He shifted from one foot to the other awkwardly, trying not to stare at her hastily closed robe and still dripping red hair. But his flushed face gave him away.

"Hang on for a second. I have to find my purse."

"Already paid for, ma'am."

"Well, I want to give you a tip," she said, glancing at the rain pouring down outside. She pressed five dollars into his hand.

He was a nice-looking young man, with dark brown hair that flopped in his eyes and was shaved close in the back. A darling little stud earring adorned his left ear. His eyes were nearly black when she could see them, for his glance shifted back and forth from a location she figured was somewhere near her neck to a space about three inches in front of her blue-lacquered toes. Her face flushed and she grabbed the collar of the robe as she pushed the door closed with her hip.

She inhaled the fragrance of the twelve blood-red roses. She'd been so wrapped up in the conference all week that she'd forgotten today was their anniversary. Joshua never forgot.

To the woman who fulfills all of my dreams. Love, Joshua.

"All but one dream, my dear," she said softly. They always had cherished the idea of having a child, but when they finally had learned that Joshua was sterile, they both had put their energies into building careers. More than once, she nearly suggested they adopt. But for Joshua, adoption would have been an admission of his own imperfection—another twist of the knife his father had thrust into his side when he was still a boy. So she dared not bring it up while Martin was still alive, and these days she seldom thought about children. Her patients, not to mention Joshua, gave her numerous opportunities to be nurturing.

The flowers looked so beautiful. Ruth poured a cup of coffee, pulled up a stool, and stared at them. Ironic, the circumstances. Martin Caliban had to die for Joshua's dream to be born.

Shortly after Joshua's mother died, Martin Caliban's business went downhill rapidly, its cash flow drained as though somebody had pulled the plug. Within six years, what had once been one of the largest car dealerships in the country was ignominiously sold off at auction.

Martin had never been able to pull himself together after Naomi's death. So he focused all the blame on his son. He never forgave Joshua for abandoning him to follow his own dreams in medicine. He ignored Joshua's accomplishments and progress while giving him false hopes of an inheritance.

"Damn Japs!" he'd say. "They lost the battle, but they won the war. How's an honest American going to compete? Now I have nothing left. But don't you worry, son. You'll be well taken care of. Your old man has stashed away a few winning tickets in a safe-deposit box for you." Over and over, he'd repeat this, waving the key like a trout fly in front of Joshua's nose.

"Don't worry, Dad, I've got all the money I need," Joshua would answer. "You know how much doctors make." But Martin Caliban would pull the key out of his pocket and lay it in the palm of his hand, stroking it with his fingers. Martin taunted Joshua, going on and on about how much money he'd stashed away, all the hard work he'd done to get it. Then the minute Joshua showed an interest in the key, Martin would yank it away giving Joshua his Chinese warlord look. "I'm *not* dead yet," he'd say. "Don't go spending all your money now before you've even got it."

Even though he desperately needed money to expand the hospital, he would rather walk on nails before he asked his father for a loan. He began to wish secretly that his father would die, and this wish perversely burdened him with guilt.

Ruth pulled on a single strand of hair—an old graduate school habit to help her concentrate. Fits of anger were the price extracted by guilt and resentment. Joshua was proof that a prodigious intelligence and deep intuition didn't guarantee immunity against Oedipal dynamics. She chuckled. Her thesis advisor would have been so wise. "Easier to see it than to be it," she'd said, warning Ruth against trying to be her own, or her spouse's, therapist.

Joshua had been out in the country on one of his rare fishing expeditions when his father finally succumbed to high blood pressure. Somehow it seemed appropriate that Martin would die of something resembling an apoplectic fit.

Joshua called Ruth from the safety of his cabin and asked her to handle the funeral. She willingly took care of everything, including the cremation Martin had wanted, but she felt fairly certain that Joshua might have begun to forgive his father if he could have participated in his final chapter. Without such closure, Joshua wasn't able to face up to later confrontations.

Two days after the service, Ruth had picked Joshua up at the airport. They went straight to the bank. Ruth never forgot Joshua's expression when he gave the safe-deposit key to the teller. He looked like a little boy passing his first nickel over the counter in a candy shop, his face full of eager, naked craving.

"Here are the final papers regarding my father's estate, and as the only heir, I'm here to open his safe-deposit box," he'd said, with obvious pride. "Here's the death certificate as well as my own birth certificate."

The teller said he'd have to speak to the bank president. Joshua winked innocently at Ruth. "It must be a real pile!" he whispered to her.

"Dr. Caliban. My name is Geoffrey Day. I'm the president of the bank. Could I ask you both to step into my office for a moment, please?" A short, balding man impeccably groomed and wearing a crisp Brooks Brothers suit smiled unctuously.

Joshua had mumbled as they followed Mr. Day into his office, "It must be too much to open up in public." Ruth had felt something was wrong right away, but held her tongue. Her negativity was perhaps a reaction to Mr. Day's lack of personal warmth. Even if he was a bank manager, did he have to be so damned ingratiating?

"My condolences at your loss," Mr. Day said. "May I offer either of you a cup of coffee or tea?"

"No thanks. We'd just like to collect the contents of the box and be on our way." Joshua's hand squeezed hers until her fingertips turned red. Waiting was not on his agenda. Joshua had hospitals to build.

"Well, I'm sorry to be the bearer of bad news so soon after your father's passing. But … uh … but there are complications." Mr. Day squirmed in the magnificent oak executive chair and fidgeted with his bifocals behind his expansive desk like a trout on the hook. Ruth remembered thinking she would have liked to have ripped those ridiculous, pretentious glasses off his face, but her job was to be a rock for Joshua, and that was what she had done.

"Complications? Aren't the papers I brought all in order?" Ruth squeezed his hand gently, but he didn't respond.

George Day squirmed some more and rocked in his seat like a little pinstriped robot—all the while holding the literal key to their future. Worse, his voice had become tinny and nasal, sounding like a mechanical toy.

"Oh yes, they most certainly are in order. Under normal circumstances, they'd be more than sufficient to release the contents of the box in question … in a situation like this, where, as you said, you are the only heir to the deceased's estate."

"What exactly, Mr. Day, is the complication?" Ruth asked, calmly.

"Well you see, Mrs. Caliban," Mr. Day had said with relief, turning away from Joshua's glare, "when the late Mr. Caliban passed away, we were forced to open the box."

Joshua had risen from his seat so fast Mr. Day's mouth had frozen in action. "You did what?" Joshua exploded, launching himself across the mahogany desk just inches from Day's face. Mr. Day's head snapped back as Joshua bellowed like a wounded bull. "If anything was touched in that box, I'll sue this bank for every penny it's worth!"

Of course he had absolutely no idea what the box contained. Nor was he aware that he'd almost pulled Ruth's arm out of its socket when he dragged her across the desktop with him.

Geoffrey Day had stuttered as he'd tried to catch his breath. "We had no choice, Dr. Caliban. The I.R.S. investigator had all the necessary papers. Your father was the sole owner of his business. No other living relative was designated as a director, his wife having passed away."

"What was it that the I.R.S. was looking for?"

Mr. Day cleared his throat. His voice was smooth and controlled. "It seems that Mr. Caliban had been using Social Security withholdings to cover his cash flow needs. Even so, he was unable to fulfill his obligations with the assets that remained when he disposed of his business. The I.R.S. put a lien on all other known assets. They're quite thorough, you know. Their investigation led them to us. We had no choice but to cooperate."

"Why wasn't I notified?" Joshua gasped, slumping back in his chair, his hand turning clammy in Ruth's.

"As I said, Dr. Caliban, we were under no obligation by law. Your father was the only authorized signatory on the card. He was the sole owner of his business."

"Is there any way we can find out how much was in the box at the time it was opened, Mr. Day?" Ruth asked.

Mr. Day straightened up and pulled at his gold-studded cuff-links. "Well, technically, I probably shouldn't be the one to divulge that information. However, it is bank policy that a senior partner of the bank be present at all such procedures in order to notarize the exact nature of the contents removed. And it was me who served as witness. I guess under these unusual circumstances and given your stature and reputation in the community, Dr. Caliban, I can bend the bank's policies just this once." He paused and cleared his throat again. "When the I.R.S. investigator opened the box, it was empty."

Joshua cupped his hands over his ears, shaking his head. His father's own insatiable thirst for gambling, not the Japanese, had defeated Martin Caliban. He had lost everything.

Ruth hadn't been able to get him to say anything the whole long way back to the house. With withdrawal or explosion as his only options, Joshua simply shut himself in.

He finally broke down that night in bed. Curled up next to her, embracing her from behind and pulling her to his chest so tightly his fingers left their prints in her shoulders, he whispered, "There ... there goes ... the hospital." She turned to him then and took him in her arms, pulling his head down to her breast. He sobbed uncontrollably, his breathing hot and moist against her skin.

She took his face in her hands and whispered back to him, crooning, her voice barely audible, "Joshua, I need you to do something for me. Something more important to me than anything else I will ever ask of you."

"What is it, sweetheart?"

"You have to let me help you build the hospital. You have to let me do it. I can, you know. You have to let me in. You can't do this by yourself."

Joshua didn't say anything, but his breathing started to slow and become more regular.

"I have money left from the insurance I got after my parents were killed in the plane crash. It really was a massive amount. My graduate school bills are all paid off. I still have money I can give to you."

She waited again, but still Joshua breathed and said nothing. "After all, let's be logical about this. If I were to die, the money would be yours anyway. And since I'm not planning on dying any time soon ... think of it this way. Maybe it would help *me* to heal more of *my* own wounds knowing that I can do this to help both of us heal others. Isn't that what we've dedicated our lives to? Isn't that why we're together?"

"I've never accepted anything from anybody in my whole life. Everything I've made, I've made for myself. I'm enough like my old man in that regard, at least," he said bitterly. "But who else can I trust, if not you? You're my darling, my sweet angel, and you know me too well. I'll think about it, but only under one condition."

"What's that, my love?"

"It will be a loan, complete with a promissory note … and I'll pay interest of a special nature."

"Oh, my noble husband, what is this interest of which you speak?" Ruth teased as Joshua softened in her arms. His tension was dissipating as his limbs twined with hers. She'd stroked the thick mane of his hair.

"Witch, tease me not. I'm falling asleep. But I'll not fall under your spell until I've exacted from you the promise that you'll take part of the money and build your clinic. We'll call it the Ruth J. Caliban Abuse Clinic. Catchy, isn't it?" Joshua managed a small laugh. "It's been your dream for as long as mine has been of the hospital. Inside it, you can build your sacred space, what do you call it?"

"*Temenos*," she whispered, her eyes stinging with tears.

"Tell me the story," Joshua murmured, drowsy.

"You remember, it's the sacred grove where adults can become like children again, free, playful, full of hope … innocent."

"We'll install a marble plaque over the door. *Lux in tenebris lucet*. 'A light shining in darkness.' That's what you are to me, Ruth."

"Joshua, you're going all romantic on me, now. I don't think I can take it. Go to sleep."

"You're a miracle worker, Ruth. You can heal me, just like you do all your patients. Take away these scars, take away my pain ... ."

"Sleep, my love."

Twelve years had passed, and now Ruth set the vase of roses, one for every year, on the breakfast table in the alcove. Out of that night of pain had been born their life's work. Joshua made good on his acceptance of her gift, and together they conceived and built both the hospital and the abuse center, and raised them into full-fledged, successful, state-of-the-art health care institutions.

She reached across the table to the wall phone and pushed one of the automatic dialing buttons. "Good morning, Dr. Caliban's office."

"Hi, Mary. How are you?"

"Ruth! Crazy, as usual. And the conference?"

"Speech went well. The rest of it pretty boring. You know what a bunch of doctors can be like ... with notable exceptions. Is Joshua free, by any chance?"

"Sorry, he's just left for lunch with a Dr. Moerae King. Can I have him call you back?"

"No. No need to bother him. Just tell him I called and thanks for the beautiful roses. I'll see him when he gets home."

"Oh! Today something special? He's so shy about these things, he rarely tells me when anything's up."

"Not to worry, Mary, it's a special day for us. He'll understand. Now, would you transfer me to Carla's line? And please let me know when you and I can get together for lunch. It's been too long since we've had a girls' day out."

"I'm penciling you in for next week as we speak. Hang on, now, dear, and I'll get you Carla." Elevator music filled the line.

"Hello. The Ruth J. Caliban Abuse Clinic. How may I help you?"

"Hi, Carla. Do me a favor, would you, and check my schedule book? I'm exhausted after this conference. If we don't have any potential jumpers on our hands, I could use a rest."

"Hold on a minute while I pull your schedule up on my screen." After a moment Carla said, "Okay, it looks good. You're in luck, Ruth. Your two o'clock cancelled and your three-thirty won't go over the edge if I reschedule."

"Terrific! Can you please get the mountain of mail I must have over to Joshua's office? I won't forget you for this, Carla. See you Monday."

For the next few hours Ruth unpacked, washed clothes, and generally got grounded again, smiling all the while. The telephone interrupted her shortly after two.

"Hello. Calibans' residence."

"Hello, Ruth, it's Moerae."

"Hi, Moerae. I'm so glad it's you! I've been on pins and needles all afternoon expecting you to call. Mary told me you and the man were out to lunch. How did you ever get an appointment so quickly? I'm dying to find out what happened! I even canceled my appointments this afternoon so I could be here in case you called."

"I know. I called the clinic and they told me you were at home. But slow down, girl, I can't answer all your questions at once." Moerae's rich, low laugh reverberated over the line.

Moerae and Ruth had been friends ever since Moerae had attended one of Ruth's seminars. She had lectured on synchronicity, and during a coffee break, Moerae had come up to Ruth.

"I have a special interest in how Jungian concepts can be applied to entire organizations as human systems," she began "Could we have lunch sometime?"

Ruth was won over immediately by Moerae's direct approach. Their first lengthy chat had taken place over *salades nicoises* and a shared bottle of Vouvray. Both admitted to a secret passion for black bottom pie and indulged, ritualistically, in a piece each. The rich chocolate pudding and meringue confection on its homey graham-cracker crust became a symbol of their confederacy. Black and white united in goodness. From then on, they'd shared numerous conference platforms and decadent lunches. Good friends and intellectual equals who could collaborate were rare.

"It went very well. We talked and I mean, we *talked*, and scratched below the surface enough that he trusts me to submit a written proposal to him. You have good taste, Ruth. I can see why you've kept him away from me all these years. He's pretty damn cute."

"Well, I said so, didn't I? Now, maybe you'll listen to me." Ruth laughed. "But, on a serious note, with all the trouble he's having with the board at C.C.A., I don't think he'll have an easy time selling it to them."

"Would you relax? You have to remember who you're talking to. I'm the *other* miracle worker, Mother Goose, and you helped teach me. And very well, I might add. You should hear yourself. You sound exactly like an anxious parent. Leave the board to me. They're like children acting out against their patriarch—big, mean ol' Daddy Joshua; and we can use that to our advantage. I have lots to tell you about all the gory details of our lunch together, but it'll have to wait. Also, I want you to read the proposal when I've drafted it, before I give it to Joshua. But I'm in a cab right now so be quick, and give me the main headlines on how your speech went down."

"Okay, I'll control my curiosity, in deference to all the help you've given me on it the last few weeks. Thanks again, by the way. You're a doll."

"Ruth Caliban, you know perfectly well I'm not fishing for compliments. Get on with your story," Moerae said chuckling.

"Well, as you know, I was nervous about it because I've had it on my mind since graduate school. I'll never forget what that old goat Withers said to me when I was in training. Remember, he was the therapist I told you about who had it in for me because I was overly fond of Jung instead of Freud? Anyway, he told me that my childhood sexual nightmares were nothing more than repressed fantasies. The nerve of him, that retrograde thinker!" Ruth laughed. "I sassed back and he accused me of being counter-dependent. I was young and full of myself, and I was so angry with him, I lost it. I said denial and projection were diseases that struck all human beings, including human beings in the helping professions as well! You can imagine how well he took that."

"Do tell, Ruth. Don't leave me in suspense."

"Are you sure I haven't told you this story already? Anyway, I vowed to find a way to help my colleagues in the field to understand how their own repressed emotions might have an effect on their patients. But you know how it is, people go into psychology in order to heal themselves, so I didn't make too many friends while I was in training."

"I told you, you were nuts to make this the subject of your talk. You're either the bravest woman I know, or the biggest glutton for punishment. So give. How did they take it?"

Ruth sighed. "Like I was a pain in their butts."

"Pretty much what we expected. And their reaction was perfectly normal. Remember the old Sufi saying, 'I never taught anyone archery who at some point did not aim their arrows at my back'."

"I have a feeling I'm going to have to remind you of that little maxim, if Joshua takes you on," Ruth said, laughing. "Do you really think he's interested?"

"There was some hesitation, especially in response to our theory that organizations go through developmental stages just like people do. And he spit out the 'personal responsibility starts at home in the boardroom' piece, but I didn't really expect him to swallow that one right away. Denial doesn't usually yield to the first assault. But yes, I think he's nibbling at the bait."

"Joshua loves a good intellectual debate." Ruth hesitated, then asked, "How did it go in the other areas?"

"The other areas? My, my, you're so delicate, my dear. Of course he asked me about my wedding ring. He hardly took his eyes off of it for the first forty minutes. I decided to take a calculated risk and gave him my lesson on Practical Sex 101."

"Oh my God, Moerae, you shock me," Ruth said in mock horror. "How did he handle it?"

"I thought he would pee in his pants! He made a rapid recovery though, making like it was the most normal thing in the world. Which it is of course. To tell you the truth, I think he was relieved to have me taken out of the sexual arena, so to speak, and, at the same time, my guess is that he started entertaining other kinds of fantasies about me. You know how men are about the two women thing. But here's something to think about: I felt so relieved by his reaction that I may have let my guard down and mentioned your first name by accident. I'm not sure he heard it. At least, he didn't respond. But it worries me. He's pretty sharp."

Ruth frowned. She didn't like working behind Joshua's back to enlist extra troops in his battle with the board, but she also knew how prideful he could be about accepting help. It was a very old story. "Don't worry," she said to Moerae. "I plan on telling him. I wanted him to form his impression of you independently."

Moerae's voice was starting to fade. "I'm afraid my phone's losing the signal."

"That's okay. I'm up to my elbows making Joshua's favorite meal for tonight and I need to get back to it."

"What are you talking about? Making his favorite meal should be easy for you by now, but you'll still have to cook something, too. I'll call you soon."

Ruth dipped her spoon into the borscht and tasted it while looking thoughtfully out the kitchen window into the yard. The rain had stopped. She brushed aside her misgivings, letting her mood lift again. The low whine of a car engine and screech of brakes startled her and her hand jerked. "Yikes," she squealed as she burned herself on the simmering pot. She glanced up at the wall clock and thought that Joshua was surprising her by getting home early. No—a knock was coming from the back door.

"Hang on a second," she yelled out over the crescendo of the 1812 Overture. She reached across the sink to turn down her portable stereo, then wiped her hands on the apron around her waist and licked a red splotch of soup off her burned arm. "Um, good, if I do say so myself." She turned down the heat under the pot roast stewing on the other burner and went to the door.

"Damn, this is just what I need." Scott MacDonald's wife Elaine waved at her through the window.

Without waiting for a hello, Elaine waltzed in. Typical, Ruth thought in exasperation.

"I was driving home and saw your car in the driveway, so I thought I'd stop in for a cup of coffee or something. Am I interrupting anything?" Elaine sang out in an obnoxiously cheerful voice.

Ruth listed all the reasonable excuses she could use to get Elaine in and out of her kitchen as fast as possible. She didn't really dislike Elaine, but since neither she nor Joshua had a lot of time to spend socially, they tended to spend what free time they had with really close friends. Besides it was painful to bear witness to Elaine's and Scott's obsessive drinking over dinner and listen to the McDonalds complain about their children and at the same time, to endure their incessant prying as to why the

Calibans didn't have any progeny of their own. Ruth was sick of having to explain why they hadn't adopted. And besides, if Elaine MacDonald was dropping by, she either had some gossip she couldn't keep to herself or she was dying to bitch about something at the hospital.

Ruth walked back to the stove and picked up the ladle. "Actually, I am preoccupied at the moment, Elaine. I hope you'll forgive me. I'm in the midst of finishing a special dinner for Joshua and me." Ruth stole a glance at Elaine and sighed when she saw Elaine's uplifted face go slack with disappointment. What the heck, Elaine might shed some light on what got Joshua so upset. "I've got a few minutes' grace period though, so grab yourself a cup of coffee. You know where everything is. Or would you prefer soda. Have whatever you want, but you'll have to get it yourself."

Elaine's foxy walnut eyes darted to the clock. She moved toward the liquor cabinet. "It's so close to happy hour, I think I'll have a pick-me-upper. That smells fab." She sniffed with her rather prominent nose up in the air.

"What's the occasion?"

Ruth stole a glance as Elaine poured a healthy dose of single malt scotch into a tall glass and nodded. She needed to divert the conversation away from where it was surely going. "I've been away at a conference all week. Didn't get home until just this morning. This will be the first chance Joshua and I will have to catch up. How're you doing?"

"You guys are such love birds," Elaine said. She held the glass up to the light and added another shot. "Don't you ever get tired of each other? Of course, if I had a hunk like yours, I'd probably wanna have dinner without a crowd more often, too."

Elaine flounced to the freezer, exuding her air of unquestioned entitlement, and stuck the glass under the automatic icemaker. She was an unabashed, completely uninhibited flirt, and as far as Ruth knew, it wasn't all talk and no action, either. It drove Scott crazy, and that of course, was Elaine's purpose.

"We're both pretty tired and stressed out these days," Ruth offered. "That probably has more to do with wanting to dine alone than getting into bed with each other."

"Yeah, I gather it was a pretty bloody meeting last night."

"There seem to be no easy ones these days," Ruth said, as non-committally as possible. Just how much did Elaine know about the meeting? It certainly would be more than she herself knew at the moment. Ruth stooped to peer in at the cake in the oven and waited for Elaine to continue.

Elaine gulped down half the glass. "Scottie told me C.C.A. almost had a palace revolt on their hands last night. The king could've been beheaded." She emptied her glass and headed back to the cabinet.

As lightly as if she'd just heard of a traffic jam on Lake Shore Boulevard, Ruth said, "The natives getting restless, are they?"

Elaine came up alongside Ruth. Stirring her drink with her diamond-laden finger, she peered nosily into the open pot while Ruth poured some cooking sherry into it. "This one's serious, Ruth," she said, her voice going nasal with what she must have thought was added drama. Ruth suppressed a giggle. "Damien wants to cut the doctors' pay by ten percent this year."

"The entire country's economy has gone sour, Elaine," Ruth replied. "Ten percent isn't going to hurt the doctors that much."

Elaine took another healthy swig. "Easy for you to say. If someone asks, 'Is there a doctor in the house?' both of you stand up. The rest of us plebeians have to struggle to make ends meet."

Ruth had heard this argument before. Poor, pathetic Elaine MacDonald. One would never know she already had so much. Brother! Although she and Joshua had plenty of things to worry about, money wasn't one of them. She couldn't really put herself in Elaine's place, and that made her feel a little sad, too. Because

---

80

of their spiritual bankruptcy, Elaine MacDonald and many financially wealthy people like her could only see themselves as victims.

"You know what they say, Elaine, money can't buy happiness."

"Yeah, but it can sure take the edge off being miserable."

The phone rang and Ruth picked it up with relief, speaking into the receiver immediately. "Hello, sweetheart. Where are ya? Yes, almost ready. How long will you be? Fifteen minutes? Great! No, we've got everything we need in the house. See you soon."

Ruth wiped her hands again on her apron and started toward the back door, hoping Elaine would take the hint. "That was Joshua. He's just pulling off the expressway. Be home in fifteen minutes. I've got to get cracking on dinner."

"How did you know that was him before you even picked up the phone?" Elaine asked. She rattled the dwindling ice cubes in her second empty glass.

"Joshua had the car phone set up so that a special button on the house phone lights up when he's calling."

"I gotta find out why my Scottie hasn't gotten his little poochie one of those toys," Elaine said, her voice slurring slightly. Ruth cringed. Elaine's husband hated being referred to as Scottie.

Elaine weaved out the door and disappeared without so much as a good-bye.

The timer went off. The chocolate anniversary cake was ready to come out of the oven. Ruth set it on the counter to cool. She reached into the kitchen drawer to get the candles she'd been saving for the cake and looked at the words on the box. They were birthday candles. A tear rolled down her cheek and she swallowed hard. Fanned by a ticking biological clock, that persistent flame of desire for a child still burned in her heart in spite of all she had done to pour her mother love in her work.

The ring of a second timer, announcing the pot roast was ready to come off the stove, startled her.

"All right, Ruth, get a grip." she whispered. The roast wasn't done yet, and she reset the timer. "Focus. Spilled milk." she said. "What needs to be done? Keep your mind on dinner, Caliban." She wiped her eyes with the back of her hand. Then she sat down next to the roses. Outside the window a bird's nest sat high in the oak tree that sheltered the greater part of the yard.

Maybe she wouldn't have made such a great mother, anyway. Nature sometimes protected people in unknowable ways. The fact that she'd never had a child might have been a blessing. Her work at the clinic brought numerous examples of how the psychic scars sustained in childhood influenced and warped their behavior as adults and even parents. Who knows? Perhaps her own horrific experiences would debilitate her as a mother. Sometimes, she still wondered if she had completely worked through the shame driven into her by her father when he used to come into her room. Late at night, he would exercise his terrible power over her, forcing her to submit to his lust and then keep silent about it.

Ruth fingered a soft rose petal then traced the stem of a rose, studded with thorns. Touching a sharp point, she came back to herself, sitting at the table, and realized that her breathing was again normal and her cheek dry.

The squeaking of the automatic garage door opener brought a broad smile to her lips.

Ruth hurried to the door. Joshua put his case down and reached for her without saying a word. He swept her into his embrace and against his chest, his lips pressing her mouth open, gently at first, then pulling at her lips and tongue.

They pulled apart for an instant, but held each other by the arms. "Hey, you," Ruth said huskily. "Did you miss me?"

"What do you think?" Joshua said, winking and then patting her behind. "Nice ... the new skirt, too. Feels like I haven't seen you in a month instead of a week. Been a hell of a time. How about you, sweetheart? God, I thought this day would never end."

Joshua broke away and pulled off his raincoat. "The storm has decided it isn't over yet. It's pouring out there, which made the traffic god-awful. Happy birthday, darling. Did you get the roses?"

"Happy birthday to you, too, sweetheart. The roses are beautiful. They arrived first thing this morning."

Joshua crossed to the stove in three giant strides. "How you can cook a pot roast that tastes and smells just like my mother's without ever having even met her is beyond me."

"I am a woman of many mysterious qualities," Ruth said, wrinkling her nose. "No peeking," she teased as he lifted the cover from the pot. "And don't burn your nose. It's not done yet. I was rather rudely interrupted in the middle of cooking it."

Joshua went into the hallway to hang his coat in the closet. "I thought you sounded in a hurry to get off the phone when I called," he yelled.

Ruth thumbed quickly through the pile of mail Joshua brought and responded as casually as possible. "Elaine dropped by to chat."

"No work tonight, woman," Joshua said, taking the pile from her and dumping it on the counter. Wrapping his arms around her bottom, he kissed her again. "Dropped by to shat would be more like it. The woman should have been a mushroom farmer, the way she loves to spread manure around."

83

"It sounded serious, Joshua. She said there was almost a palace revolt. 'The king could have been beheaded.' Those were her exact words." Ruth leaned her head back to look at him.

From his briefcase he pulled out a memo and passed it to her. "The turkeys had the nerve to hand me an ultimatum."

She read the memo silently. When she looked up, Joshua was standing at the liquor cabinet, holding a bottle of Jack Daniels in one hand and reaching for a glass with the other. Damn. A hard day and a glass of the hard stuff was not a good combination. "I've got a bottle of our favorite wine to go with dinner," she said.

He held up his half-full glass. "It's okay, I just want to take the edge off. It hasn't been the easiest of weeks. You want anything from here?"

She shook her head. The memo disturbed her. Confrontations such as these stretched him. And when Joshua was stretched, he reached for the bottle for help, not to her. His excuse would be that she had enough to handle with the clinic without having to be his therapist, too. But Ruth knew it was also because he wanted to be a big boy and take care of his own problems.

"No, I'll stick with the wine," she said. "It's in the bucket. So what do you think this means?" She held out the memo.

"It means they're pissed about the ten percent cut. Shit, I wish they would invent a corkscrew that you don't need a PhD to use!"

Ruth watched him struggle without offering to help, trying unsuccessfully to mask her irritation. "I can see that! From what Elaine said, it's perfectly obvious why they'd resent having their resources cut back, especially without being privy to the decision. After all, that's what made you the most angry, isn't it? No, Joshua, what I meant was, what can you do about it? They're acting like it's your fault."

"Here," he said, handing her a glass. "Chardonnay à la cork."

Ruth placed her hands on her hips, her legs slightly splayed. "Joshua, give. You're going to have to tell me what the hell went on in that meeting before I'll be able to relax enough to enjoy dinner. And I want dinner to be relaxing."

Joshua put up his hands and feigned protecting himself. "Okay, okay, Amazon Woman, but I don't want to spoil our meal with a gory postmortem. Not to mention dessert, à la bed!"

"I can't wait," she said, fluttering her walnut eyelashes. "Just give me the headlines. But don't leave anything out for the sake of brevity, because I want to know what we're up against." She gestured toward the breakfast nook. "Let me turn the stove down and we can sit over there so I can keep an eye on the roast."

Joshua settled into his chair and leaned back, running his fingers through his silvery hair. Ruth listened as much to how Joshua recounted the story as to what he was telling her. Stiff body, head set deep on his shoulders, nervous arm movements, and the way he punctuated his thoughts with sharp jabs of his hands showed his anger. But he was justifiably angry, as far as she could tell, and thank God he didn't seem obsessed with the need to get even with anyone. If she could coax him into confiding his fears, she could relieve some of the pressure. Given time and a good session in bed, she could take the sting out of his wounded pride.

"The good news is, I think I've found a consultant who can really help."

Ruth leaned forward smiling. "Oh, yeah? Tell me what she said."

A knowing smile immediately crossed Joshua's face, followed by a deep belly laugh. "You imp! I *knew* I heard her refer to you by name. Did you set me up, woman?"

She crossed her arms and lifted her chin in a feigned hurt expression. "Would I do that? We met at a conference and hit it off. Even helped me prepare the paper I gave this week. She's very interested in the application of Jungian theory to organizations. I wanted your first impression to be unclouded by our relationship. She called this afternoon to tell me how excited she was to have met you and to have the opportunity to possibly work with you. I'm glad to hear that you liked her."

"To be honest, I was more impressed than I thought I'd be. I can barely handle the one psychologist already in my life." He gave her his own look of mock seriousness as he put his empty whiskey glass in the sink. "Let's eat. The smell of that pot roast is driving me nuts."

Ruth decided for the time being not to worry about whether the wind blowing off Lake Michigan carried storm clouds or the sweet smell of success. She was glad Joshua wasn't refilling his glass. The rest of the evening will be serene.

"Go get the album and I'll dish out the borscht," she said.

Joshua placed the album on the table, walked slowly up behind her, and wrapped his arms protectively around her waist. Bending his head, he kissed her on the neck just below her ear. Without turning, Ruth tilted her head so their lips could meet, then twisted around completely and stroked her fingers through his beard, delighted in the shiver that ran through his body.

Ruth looked at the hand-knit cover she'd made and smiled. They'd started the album the night after they'd decided to use some of Ruth's inheritance to propel C.C.A. into the big leagues. In it they'd pasted all the "baby pictures" of their growing, tandem organizations. No one else had ever seen it.

Between courses, they looked through the album. The original suite of offices on the second floor of the professional building had spread to include the main campus on the outskirts of Chicago. Satellite offices in Florida and Arizona offered care for elderly Chicagoans fleeing the winter cold.

"When the twins" as Joshua referred to the two new satellite facilities "were born, the board resisted it," he said through a mouthful of gravy-laden potatoes.

Ruth nodded. "Could I ever forget? Until you pointed out to them that they could retire down there, too, along with their patients. And this one was a real brawl," Ruth said, pointing to a picture of the inner-city clinic that served Chicago's growing underprivileged masses. "The bank wouldn't fund the building because they thought it wasn't a good business venture."

Joshua groaned. "Yeah, I remember that one particularly well. We had to convince the guys to personally guarantee the loan. But God bless 'em, they finally gave in."

"Sometimes I feel so hopeless, Joshua," she said, stroking the picture of the Ruth J. Caliban Abuse Clinic with her fingertips as if it were a beloved face. "For every soul we help, there are thousands more who live out their days in loneliness and pain. I know now hard it is to be whole and healthy inside."

Joshua stroked his beard. "God, have we grown. From fourteen doctors sharing office space to an army of almost a thousand. Eight thousand families draw their sustenance from us, Hon, and one hundred times that number come as patients."

Ruth nodded and freed her ponytail from its band.

Joshua closed the album and leaned back, patting his full stomach. "I've got a full morning tomorrow. What say we clean up and hit the sack?"

"Tomorrow's Saturday. It's Martha's day to come in to clean the house, so we can leave the dishes. Don't you want some dessert?" she asked, pointing to the chocolate cake covered in whipped cream. "I baked it myself." Joshua smiled. "Bring a piece upstairs. If any crumbs drop in your lap, I'll lick them off."

"You're incorrigible!" Ruth exclaimed.

Slowly, deliberately, keeping her eyes on Joshua, Ruth dropped a huge dollop of extra whipped cream on the slice she'd cut for him. As she lifted the plate with the piece of cake she'd cut, Ruth licked her lips. The extra whipped cream was already starting to dribble down the side.

Six

As soon as he entered the room, Joshua shivered. A musty smell like unwashed sweat pants lay undisguised under a recent application of hospital disinfectant. A once brilliant bouquet of blooms sat drooping in the corner by the bed. Damn. Joshua believed people meant well by sending flowers to cheer their friends and relatives, but their very fragility only managed to underscore life's impermanence.

Mr. Wong sat with his head slumped loosely on his barrel chest, looking like a discarded puppet, its strings severed. When Joshua came in, he looked up with tear-filled eyes and shrugged. "Bingo," he said softly.

Joshua put his hand on the older man's stooped shoulder. "I'm so sorry," he began. "I'm so terribly sorry."

He thought of the kiss he'd given Mrs. Wong moments before opening her up and a lump of sadness mixed with anxiety arose from his chest to his throat. He always felt some grief when any of his patients died, but these days, his grief was constantly accompanied by apprehension. No matter how heroic or skillful his effort, the guillotine of liability for the patient's death hung over his head.

"No, no, Doc. You did everything you could," Mr. Wong said. Had age made the old man clairvoyant or just simply more intuitive about other people's thoughts? Mr. Wong blinked away the tears welling up in his eyes. "Her number just came up a moment ago. I haven't even called the nurse yet." Mr. Wong turned back to stroking long strands of silver hair away from his wife's forehead.

Mr. Wong had propped his wife's head up on the pillows so she could catch a last glimpse of the flowers growing outside her window. Joshua was transfixed by the serene expression on the old lady's face smoothing out the fine lines that had creased her skin. Her eyes were closed tenderly as if she were only asleep. Joshua hoped with all his soul that her last words to him had come true, that she had died with love in her heart. Out of habit, he leaned over to place his stethoscope on her chest.

"She really liked you, Doc. Even told me you'd kissed her before the operation. Meant a lot to her. She kept nagging me this mornin' to call you so she could talk to you. I told her you were a busy man, it bein' a Saturday and everything. So she made me write down this letter to read to you." Mr. Wong fumbled in his coat pocket and withdrew a crumpled paper folded in half. Stopping to fish his handkerchief out of another pocket, his shoulders shook so much that his hands trembled. "A letter she never finished." Mr. Wong broke into sobs.

Joshua reached for the letter but Mr. Wong stopped him. "No, Doc, I promised I would read it to you, and you know my wife. If I don't keep that promise, she won't let me rest in peace." Wiping his eyes and blowing his nose again, Mr. Wong began:

Dear Joshua, Henry told me I should call you doctor, but I told him that when a man touched my heart the way you did, I can call him whatever I like. Thank you for the window seat. I feel like I am back home in my own garden. I love flowers. They're just like people. Once the seed takes hold, then we have to water the seedlings, pull the weeds, and make sure they get plenty of warmth. Otherwise they don't have room to sprout their wings.

Henry stopped to wipe his eyes, then began again:

There ain't nothing that doesn't grow better with love. Of course, you already know that, from all the hearts you've fixed up. I told Henry to send you a copy of a little poem I wrote after the first time you operated on me. It will have to do for the tip I promised you.

Henry paused for another second to wipe his nose. Had Henry noticed that Mrs. Wong had changed her letter to the past tense?

Remind him to send it if he forgets. You know how some men can be about stuff like poetry. I also wanted to thank you for being my handsome prince. No need to worry, I told Henry myself. It helped me to nap in peace. I only wish …

Henry stopped cold, looked up and shrugged his shoulders. There was nothing more to read.

"I only wish," Joshua said, finishing for her, "that I'd taken off my mask to kiss her."

A quiet shuffling announced the arrival of Peter Albert and the floor's head nurse. They stood side by side at the door.

The nurse began, "I'm sorry, Dr. Caliban. I wasn't here when Mrs. Wong passed away. I was busy with another patient. We're short-staffed today. One of our people is out with the flu and the other had to leave early to take a professional development seminar."

"That's okay," Joshua said softly. "There's nothing we could've done. Mrs. Wong died peacefully."

Henry nodded.

Peter put his clipboard down on the bed, placed one hand on Joshua's shoulder and the other on Mr. Wong's. "Is there anything I can do?"

The image of the last time his father had kissed him on the day his mother was diagnosed with brain cancer popped into his mind. He covered Peter's hand with his own. "It's just that in all these years, I've never gotten used to death."

"You're not supposed to," Peter said.

Joshua straightened his shoulders. "I have to prepare for my meeting with Damien," he said in a low voice to Peter. "Can you arrange to have Mrs. Wong moved downstairs, and then stop by my office right after?"

"Since the day we were married, Doc," Henry said, "I ain't ever let her go to sleep without kissin' her goodnight. Even when she was in the hospital before, I kissed her when I left at night and the first thing I saw her in the mornin'. What am I gonna do now Doc? What am I gonna do without her?" Without getting up from his chair, Henry wrapped his arms around Peter's waist.

Mr. Wong's chest heaved as the nurse pulled the bed sheet over his wife's face. "Mr. Wong, we have to move your wife to another room. If you like, you can help transfer her to a gurney and then you and Dr. Albert can take her downstairs together," Joshua offered. "Then you can kiss her good-bye one more time."

"Downstairs" was hospital code for the morgue. Even though most of the other surgeons delegated the task to a nurse, Joshua usually accompanied his patients. He relinquished this responsibility only because he was anxious about the meeting with Damien.

Peter ran his pudgy fingers over his mocha colored towhead and grabbed his clipboard from the end of the bed. "Sure, I'll see you in a few minutes."

Easing out of the room, Joshua looked back one more time, then left.

He welcomed the long walk back to his office. He took the outside route, hoping the cool breeze coming off the lake would clear out some of the turmoil ripping away at his mind. Besides, if he were lucky, he could avoid running into one of his colleagues out here—especially on a Saturday. The empty hole in his stomach left no room for forced smiles or camaraderie.

In his office he found Mary, valiantly attempting to create some semblance of order out of the chaos on top of his desk. No real surprise—she spends almost every Saturday trying to help him "catch up a little." He had long ago given up on trying to convince her that this was a terrible way to spend her Saturdays—that her health was more important.

"Monkey see, monkey do," was all she said in response to his arguments. The woman was damned obstinate. And he couldn't help feeling guilty for her sacrifice, even though she swore it meant more for her to know she'd made a little more space for him, facing the next week with a clear desk.

Knows me like a book, he thought, as she prepared him a cup of hot coffee, stirring the last of the three sugars into it and waiting for him to sip it noisily before she spoke.

"Hope that's strong enough for you, Dr. Caliban. How you can tolerate that forty-weight sweet brew is beyond my understanding. You must have learned it in medical school."

"It takes a strong man to drink a strong brew, my dear. Thank you very much for indulging me," he said, managing a small smile.

Mary pulled the pencil out from its usual position between the thick waves of her silver-grey hair and grabbed her clipboard. "Well, you look as if you could use it this morning. You're looking tired. Want to talk about it?"

Joshua slid past her into his inner office and collapsed into his oversized shiny black leather chair. He leaned back and took a deep breath. "We lost one this morning." Mary waited patiently in the moment of silence that followed. Then Joshua's eyes met hers.

"Mrs. Wong. She passed away just a few minutes ago. I wish I had been there."

"Ah. She's the one you brought back from the brink a few years ago, right?"

Joshua nodded.

Mary tilted her dark chocolate eyes away from Joshua's gaze. "Were there any … uh, complications?"

"Complications? No, at least none that I'm aware of. It was pretty much routine. I appreciate your asking, Mary."

Mary hesitantly reached out to touch him, stopped, and nodded.

The knot of anxiety constricting in his heart had eased up a little. Bless her, she always got her point across without having to spell it out. "I wonder if I should've raised the issue of an autopsy with Mr. Wong, though." His voice trailed off.

But a moment later, Joshua sat up in his chair and shrugged off this last nagging doubt. "So what's in that quagmire today?"

Mary transferred her pencil back to its usual position and thumbed through the pile of pink message slips stuck on her clipboard as expertly as a bank teller fanning a stack of new bills. "Nothing that needs your immediate attention. Dr. King called to thank you for lunch. She said to tell you she might be able to get her proposal to you much sooner than she'd thought."

"The way the alligators are snapping these days, I can use all the help I can get," Joshua said, wincing at the memory of the board meeting earlier in the week. "What did you think of her?"

"We only had a few minutes to chat," replied Mary, "but I liked her. She felt—you know—real." She looked away and fanned the pile of slips again. "I gather it was pretty bloody in there Thursday night?"

Joshua smiled when she finally looked up. "You're a wily old woman, Mary, and you don't fool me for a minute fooling with that pile of paper. Jesus, that meeting didn't end until just as you were leaving and I was too busy yesterday to fill you in. You must have better sources of information than I do. Someday you'll have to tell me how you do it."

Mary dropped the papers on his desk, put her hands on her curvy hips and lifted her squared chin proudly. "We women have our ways, you know."

She winked and picked up her clipboard again. "Let's see. We got another complaint in the mail about how cold the air conditioning is in the administration building on the weekends. That's the third one this month. I passed it on to Mr. Rees. Oh, and that reminds me, Mrs. Caliban just called. She said to remind you she put your sweater in your carry bag. And Mr. Rees called to say he's in his office. You can drop over at any time. He'll be in all morning." Mary looked over her gilded bifocals at Joshua. "I'll be catching up on the rest of the mail this morning. Do you need anything for your meeting with him?"

"Bring me his personnel folder, will you please, Mary?" He paused, cleared his throat and swallowed a gulp of coffee. "And thanks for the therapy session."

Mary raised her neatly plucked eyebrows and smiled softly. "You'll get my bill in the mail. All joking aside, it sounds pretty serious if you want his file."

Joshua stretched back into his chair. He wasn't sure he believed in his own words. "There's no doubt in my mind that the situation is pretty bloody—and could get worse. But I think we can stave off a total massacre. I just want to make sure I have all the ammo I'm going to need."

He thumbed through Damien's file. The worst thing was that he didn't know if he could save Damien or not. Peter walked in and held up the coffee pot to offer Joshua a refill. "There's no rest for the weary, is there?"

"Weary with worry." Joshua shoved his empty cup across the desk with his left hand while he reached into his bottom desk drawer with his right.

"Been hitting those worry beads pretty hard lately, haven't you?" Peter asked.

"Just a little Valium, that's all. I'm not looking forward to my meeting with Damien. And Mrs. Wong's dying hit me harder than I would've expected. Did you get her downstairs for me?" Joshua stretched across his desk for the cup Peter held out to him and swallowed the pill in one gulp before Peter could see what it really was.

Peter's hazel eyes squinted just slightly, crinkling around the edges. The nostrils of his rounded nose twitched momentarily. "Yes, I had Mr. Wong help me move her to the morgue. I also took the liberty of testing his willingness to approve a limited autopsy. I hope that's okay with you."

"It's more than okay. I'm greatly relieved!" Joshua reflected, "Once again, you seem to be able to read my thoughts. After I left today, I'd actually considered broaching the subject with Mr. Wong myself. What did he say?"

Peter sat on the couch next to Joshua's desk. "He was very gracious about it. Told me that he and Mrs. Wong used to do it themselves on his father's farm whenever a cow died for no apparent reason. His main concern was whether or not she'd be able to wear her favorite dress to the wake. It seems they made promises to one another about what they would wear when they were buried so they could recognize each other in heaven."

The two men swallowed coffee in tandem.

"Their devotion to each other is rare these days, isn't it?" Peter said.

"It's a beautiful thing to witness. They were so lucky. Just like me and Ruth. Well, who's going to do the cutting?"

"I bumped into Ross on the way up, and he offered to do it himself. He'll get you the results by noon today."

"Well, well. Miracles never cease," Joshua said with a huff. "Is this the same Ross Benson, chief of pathology, who, just a couple of days ago, was personally representing the pack of wolves at my throat? Don't tell me he's sacrificing his Saturday morning for my benefit."

He inhaled a mouthful of coffee and swilled it before continuing, "You know, Ruth is right. She's told me a hundred times that just because I'm a surgeon doesn't mean I can understand the workings of the human heart when it comes to feelings. I'm just a goddamned body mechanic."

Peter uncrossed his legs, leaned forward and rested his hands on his muscular thighs. "Don't sell yourself short, boss." And don't sell Ross short, either. The jury hasn't returned a verdict on that meeting yet."

Joshua nodded. "So you say. Well, accept my thanks for handling that, Peter. I'll rest easier knowing what happened to Mrs. Wong." Joshua wiped his mouth and stroked his beard thoughtfully. "Now then, since we've broached the subject, tell me what you found out about the scene the other night, Mr. Colombo?"

"It's serious, but the bottom line is, I don't think it's a no-win situation. Don't ask me who the ringleaders are. They already think I'm your mole so nobody will talk to me. Gut instinct says the really bad blood is localized and probably not malignant. It can be contained. I also feel there's some sympathy for your side."

"So my suspicions were correct. The ringleaders *were* Scott MacDonald and Paul Blake. Paul's a snake in the grass—he never said a word during the entire board meeting. He let everyone else do his poisonous talking for him." Joshua slapped his thigh.

Peter's face remained stoic.

Joshua shook his head. "I know. I know. You ain't talking. And remind me never to play poker with you. What else you got?"

Peter locked his chunky hands and flexed his fingers. "The mob is in pain. The rest of them are ripe for being led astray. And it isn't just the physicians. I talked to Kathy a bit after you left the O.R. yesterday. She says if the docs don't bite the bullet this year, the rest of the staff will be demoralized. The pay freeze last year hit them hard. Here's how she put it: 'doctors losing ten percent isn't any worse than us struggling to make ends meet without a raise.'"

Joshua threw his arms up in exasperation as his voice went up a notch in pitch and volume. "Is every room in this building bugged or am I the only one who doesn't know what's going on around here? How does Kathy know what's being discussed in a *closed* board meeting where I'm so clueless, I get blind-sided!"

The look on Peter's face prompted Joshua to raise a hand indicating he was still under control. "It's okay, it's okay," he said. "I'll cool off again. I'm just pissed as holy hell about being left out of the loop."

"That ambush was created off campus," Peter said quickly. "And you handled it so beautifully, I'm sure it won't happen again. You have to remember that this place is just like a small town, Joshua. Things get passed through the grapevine and all over the vineyard before they sink back down to the roots."

Joshua closed his eyes and took a deep breath. "All right. I'm calm now. I know you're trying to keep us on track. What else did you find out?"

Peter paused and touched his finger to the tip of his nose. "Kathy actually made several helpful—and insightful—observations. She said if the doctors would only get their acts together, it would help a lot. Like paying more attention to patient scheduling, cutting down on so many cancellations, keeping patient records up to date, and limiting their golf greens consultation meetings. It would set a good example for the rest of the staff.

"The pay cut only scratches the surface—our staff just can't tolerate the old physician-layman double standard we've promoted for generations. We simply have to pull our prima donnas into line. It's killing morale and it can't be any good for the overall financial picture. Many of the policies we need are already in place—but if we don't enforce them, we lose credibility with the staff. We have to put some teeth into the rules—from the top down."

Joshua winced, his cheeks pushed upward by a forced smile. "I know you're right, Peter. And I should be grateful to Kathy for being so straightforward about it. Do you want to hear something ironic? It's exactly what Damien's been urging me to do for months. He's been a pain in the ass about making the board police itself, take responsibility for its own. And I'll admit, I've been guilty, too. I've gotten way behind on logging in my patient records and I know perfectly well that slows down the billing. It makes us vulnerable for fines if our charts get audited, and it jeopardizes patient safety with incomplete records."

Peter grinned broadly, again crinkling his smoothly shaved baby face. "I'm sure you took Damien's advice with your usual equanimity."

"Naturally. I was as defensive as any one of those turkeys in the meeting the other day. Right off the bat, I said, 'doctors are professionals! You can't treat us like children!'" Then he added with a self-conscious laugh, "In my own defense, I have to say I felt ashamed after the fact. But I wasn't going to let Damien know it."

"I know you believe in what I'm about to say," Peter began, flattening the corners of his curled full lips. "*All* of our people are human beings, and they deserve to be treated with equal respect. It doesn't matter if we're talking about an orderly or a janitor, a nurse or a lab technician, or the chief of surgery. We cannot afford double standards. That's as unethical as crooked bookkeeping. In other words, we can't afford to tolerate preferential treatment of management, especially compared with treatment of our staff. If we expect everyone employed at C.C.A. to act professionally, it's up to us at the top to define what that means and live by those standards."

Joshua nodded and wagged his finger at Peter. "For a little guy, you certainly have big balls. You're starting to sound like Damien. That reminds me, I've got to see him in a few minutes. I could use hearing some good news. You wouldn't by any chance happen to have any, would you?"

Peter rose and began to pace, a habitual gesture when he was about to get to his point. "Nobody likes the idea of a pay cut, myself included. But I'm beginning to wonder if the real issue isn't that we docs are just basically suspicious of anything we don't understand. Not only do they *not* teach us the business end of medicine in med school, but they teach us never to admit that we don't understand something—especially to non-physicians! And Damien's secretive and—forgive me if I'm blunt—self-righteous style of doing things just makes it worse."

Joshua smiled. "Bluntness is one of your most endearing qualities."

Peter put his hands on his love handles and nodded. "I'll remind you of that some day. Anyway, it truly widens the gulf between 'us' and 'them.' The docs need to trust, they need to know that the cut is necessary to strengthen the organization. But I don't think they'll hear it from Damien—that's not his style."

He paused, paced a few more steps, and looked straight into Joshua's steel-grey eyes. "Damien won't like it, but I propose we hire an independent audit of our financial procedures. It could go a long way toward closing the gap of our mutual mistrust."

Joshua started to rise, bit his lip, and sat down. "Damn it! We've already got the biggest accounting firm in town auditing our books. What more do they want?"

Peter held out his open palms and shrugged his narrow shoulders. "Simply saying *'independent'* audit will get their attention. They need to hear that proposal coming from one of us on the inside."

Joshua grabbed a pencil and twirled it rapidly between his powerful fingers. "You've thought this out, I presume?" Then before Peter could answer, "Of course you have, who am I talking to? You've never brought any half-baked idea or suggestion to me."

"Let me do this. All I need is a modest consultant budget, and a lighter caseload for the next couple of weeks." He grinned as he continued, "without affecting my bogie, of course!" He laughed out loud, but before Joshua could even respond, he added, "And I want you to assign Ross and Roger as my co-committee members. *And* give us complete access to all records."

"No cut in pay! Carte blanche! Is that all?"

"And no preliminary feedback to you. That has to be absolutely clear to the other board members."

Joshua tapped his hands on his chest and opened wide his deep-set eyes. "Are you implying that even I am a suspect, Mr. Colombo?"

Peter responded before realizing that Joshua was playing with him. "We want to avoid anyone suspecting the effort or me. I'm so close to you, they'll naturally expect some duplicity. And any idea coming from me must clearly not appear to be influenced by you—not in the least."

Knowing that he had already won his case, Peter turned at the door and said, "When will you propose it to the board?"

"At next week's closed meeting. I'll feel out Damien right now and let you know when I've got Ross and Roger on line. Then you can go ahead and get your consultants. Unless, of course, you've already got them." Joshua laughed.

"Just one," Peter laughed as well. "Good luck with Damien. Feel free to give me a call over the weekend if you need me. Otherwise, I'll see you Monday."

As Peter disappeared through the door, Joshua gathered his papers and began to stride from the office himself. Halfway to the door, he snapped his fingers, remembering his sweater. Damien's office was in the administration building that everyone called "The Freezer." A broad, open space of concrete separated it from the rest of the organization. It was that way not by design but by necessity, for C.C.A.'s rapid and undisciplined growth had demanded expansion of facilities and functions to accommodate it. Unfortunately, the literal separation between the complexes mirrored the ideological gulf between their occupants so well. There was never enough room.

"I'll be at Damien's office if you need me," Joshua said to Mary as he walked by her desk. "Ross Benson may come looking for me. Please ask him to wait if he can."

"I'll be here when you get back. Good luck."

Joshua crossed the open yard and, as he came up to the front door of the administration building, Allison Bridges, one of the on-duty nurses that morning on Mrs. Wong's floor, fell into step with him.

"That's a good idea," she said, pointing a crooked finger at the sweater draped over his arm. "It can get as cold as the morgue in here on the weekend."

"Not enough bodies in here on the weekend to keep the temperature up," Joshua said. When the building was full, the body heat generated was enough to keep most people reasonably comfortable. Damien's research had shown that keeping the temperature constant, rather than adjusting it up or down to adapt to the number of bodies in the building, saved money.

Even if only on the weekend. Joshua and Damien had argued about it several times, since complaints from the patients came to Joshua's office first.

"It does save us a lot of money not to turn the AC off on the weekends. Where're you headed?" Joshua asked nonchalantly as he held the door open for her.

She opened her shopping bag, exposing a yoga pillow and a sweater. "We've got a stress-management session this morning as a part of our wellness program."

"I sure could use some of that myself," Joshua responded as they got on the elevator. His spontaneous admission sent a wave of anxiety through his stomach. Was he going to be prey to these shifts of emotions all day, even after his meeting with Damien was over? Those tablets he'd just swallowed should have evened things out a bit more for him by now. "I've been meaning to sit in on that program for the longest time but never seem to find the time."

"It's mostly nurses, some other staff, and a lot of patients." A half-smile parted her magenta lips. "Most of the doctors are usually too busy."

The elevator stopped and Joshua held the door open. "Busy docs are good for business. Have a good session."

As she stepped into the corridor, Allison cocked her head to one side and nodded.

Joshua juggled his papers under his arm as he pulled on the sweater. The elevator chugged upward and he wryly noted that the sweater might not be needed. A confrontation with Damien could well generate enough emotional heat to make the sweater unnecessary. The elevator door opened and Joshua walked down the hallway towards Damien's office. He wished he'd asked Mary to call ahead. He didn't want to surprise Damien, even though he knew he'd be expected.

Joshua stopped outside the door to Damien's outer office, closed his eyes, filled his lungs with air and released it slowly. And again. Peter's presence had made him self-conscious, but now he wished he had a grabbed a few more tablets to have in his pocket. Nevertheless, he knew he could assume the appearance of a man in complete control of his faculties on sheer willpower alone—no matter *what* the circumstances. Ruth had told him so. Peter had as much as told him so. He had trained himself all his life to be the picture of confidence, a man who could handle anything.

His only doubt at the moment concerned Damien. If Damien ever got wind of the memo that Joshua had found at the head of the oak table in the boardroom, he'd personally do whatever it would take to see that heads would roll.

Holy mother, let the copy he'd stuffed in his bag be the only one left.

Seven

Damien Rees waved to the guard as he swung his big black Lincoln into the parking garage. He loved his car. He loved its ostentatious size—its excessive power. He especially loved how it responded. An easy dial of one finger turned its wheels; a slow, delicate pressure on the brake eased it to a stop. And it was quiet. He glanced in the rear-view mirror at the spare tire that sat like a bubble on top of the trunk. He smiled and flipped a bird. How delicious that all those assholes in the "Doctors' Club" hated that he could afford his own "Jew Canoe" with its built-in toilet seat. Damn shame his father wasn't alive to see him driving such a car.

Damien loved all of his material possessions. He'd just had so little for most of his life. At the top of the list was his computer. Unlike a human being, one could negotiate its inner secrets without getting nasty emotional reactions. A computer might be temperamental if one didn't give it the right commands, but it wasn't personal. It never got pissed of, never talked back. It didn't die and leave one to grieve. Give it an order and, in the blink of an eye, your wish was its command.

José, the cashier at the hospital cafeteria, flashed Damien a bright smile as he entered: "Hi, Mr. Rees."

He didn't need to look at Damien's tray as he punched numbers into the register at the food counter. The entries were always the same. An orange juice, a plain yogurt, and one coffee with a small container of real, one-hundred percent cream that the cafeteria kept in stock just for Damien.

Damien nodded at José. Pretending to scan the headlines of the folded newspaper on his tray, he treated himself to a furtive glance at José's washboard abs and biceps rippling under his white shirt. The boy had been working out.

Damien nodded again when José asked if he wanted a double sack to carry his coffee and yogurt upstairs. José's cheerful observance of his morning ritual made Damien's day, almost as much as he enjoyed checking out the high roundness of the younger man's ass. A staff member's respectful familiarity made him feel like he belonged.

"Calls me Mister," thought Damien with a trace of humor. "Wonder what he'd call me if I really got to know him?"

Inwardly, Damien had to laugh at himself for finding comfort in such small human interactions as his morning routine with José. Life would be a different if he commanded the same kind of camaraderie with the medical staff, especially the docs. But they always considered themselves to be out of his league, and they never missed an opportunity to let him know it. Joshua was the only physician who'd ever treated Damien as an equal.

Alone in the elevator, Damien flashed back on his decade with Joshua. They met as two bored guests at a party thrown by "respectable drug lords," a term they used to refer to the pharmaceutical reps relentlessly schmoozing them. In no time, they discovered a common love for Jack Daniels and a disdain for the humorless religious gatherings they each had endured as youths. Inevitably, their conversation drifted to discussing their respective health care businesses. And to his credit, Joshua first recognized the potential in C.C.A. buying Damien's string of nursing homes.

Through a series of discreet meetings, their relationship developed quickly and they plotted a new course for C.C.A. Joshua expressed his faith in Damien by saying he had found the "other half" of his own equation—the missing component that could make C.C.A. work as a business. And Damien was more than flattered; he respected Joshua's generosity in giving him credit for abilities to do what he himself couldn't.

Their discretion was rewarded handsomely. The competition was taken by surprise when Care Corporation of America announced its purchase of Damien's small chain of nursing homes. Combining their expertise and facilities, they designed a marketing campaign that showcased Joshua's cherished philosophy: providing "cradle-to-grave" care. Consequently C.C.A. quickly captured a larger share of the market.

It wasn't long before Damien grew to respect Joshua's broad intuitive vision, even though it was fed by an intelligence that was predominantly emotional. Joshua praised Damien's precision, his analytical, mathematical mind and his extraordinary mastery of digital technology.

Damien was proud of their achievement and kept a photograph in his office of Joshua and himself shaking hands on the deal. It was a constant reminder of how far the son of one of Al Capone's hired guns had come. But Joshua Caliban was still one of them. And the good doctor certainly wouldn't be a happy camper this morning.

Damien flicked his office light switch with an elbow before setting his briefcase with its precious cargo on his desk. He looked around and sighed with pleasure. His secretary was doing her job. The credenza holding his coffee pot and cups looked as immaculate as an O.R. instrument table. The mugs were made of glass instead of styrofoam. Pencils sharpened to a fine point stood handsomely at attention in a black acrylic holder. A white-gloved finger run along the edge of the walnut bookshelf wouldn't pick up a speck of dust.

Except for one photograph of his mother and the one of Joshua and Damien on his desk, nothing of his personal life intruded on his professional world. He couldn't count the number of times he'd told Joshua a stuffed dead fish just didn't cut it in a physician's office.

"Easiest thing in the world, giving other people medicine," he muttered. But he didn't know one doctor who could take a dose of his own.

A fleeting pang of anxiety stabbed at his stomach, but he brushed it aside and gulped a mouthful of yogurt. This was no time to give in to fear. He stroked the screen of his computer monitor as it lit up, calming him immediately. The world inside his computer was pure and logical and predictable, a realm of mathematical absolutes. Ones and zeroes. Black and white. No shades of gray.

Gray—the color of bleakness. Bleak—the very picture of Damien's childhood. Thirteen-year-old Damien suffered sexual abuse at the hands of his stepfather. He still blamed the cop who got a medal for killing his father. Good thing the sick bastard landed in a mental institution for abusing the boy. Otherwise, Damien was still certain that he would have made his own headlines as a teenage murderer.

He was thrown out on his own when his mother died from inhaling asbestos at a horrible job she held just to try and earn enough money to send him to medical school. He felt orphaned—abandoned. But now it seemed ironic to Damien as he swallowed the last of his orange juice: If his mother hadn't died, would he have discovered management school and his natural talent for making money?

The spreadsheets flickering on the screen called Damien back to the present. He rubbed his fingers through his thinning brown hair and wondered how long had he been lost in reverie. He blinked and stared at the numbers. Damn! Am I the only one who can look at these financials and see that there's still plenty of money to be made? Why can't the physicians who calmly monitor a patient's vital signs fluctuating within an acceptable range see that the highs and lows in C.C.A.'s cash flow were within a similar normal range? The slightest blip in the curve seemed to bring most of the doctors to the brink of cardiac arrest.

But not Joshua Caliban—he was driven by his vision and comforted by previous success in weathering tough times through the years. His vision and foresight were undeniably awesome, but often uncontrollable. That's why Damien and Joshua made a damn good team. Damien's organizational skill and obsessive attention to systems and details could channel Joshua's way-too-forward thinking.

The problem with the other docs was that they had no memories of anything that couldn't capture their interest. This galled Damien to his core. If they ever had acknowledged his contributions to their precious livelihood, they couldn't remember it now. But one day—maybe soon—they will see. Revenge would taste even sweeter for the waiting.

Damien's head snapped erect when Joshua knocked on the open door as he walked in. "Hi, Damien. Why am I not surprised to find you hunched over your monitor at this hour of the morning? Are you ever separated from that damn computer?", he laughed.

Damien waved with his left hand as his right continued to dance on the 10-key number pad. "Be with you in a minute. I'm just cleaning up some files. Grab yourself a cup." He nodded toward the ebony credenza that matched his desk.

"It never ceases to amaze me how tidy you keep this place," Joshua said as he poured himself a cup. "It's downright Spartan! My place looks like the barracks from hell. You'd never be able to function."

"Well, that's the difference between you and me," Damien mumbled without looking up.

Joshua stirred instant creamer into his cup. "Want one?"

"No thanks. I've already had my morning fix. I got started really early. I just wanted to double-check my numbers on the pay cut issue before we talked," Damien said, finally swiveling to face Joshua.

Joshua settled into the armchair beside Damien's desk. "What's it looking like?"

Damien fingered the scar that ran across his chin, signaling to Joshua that something's making him nervous, but he squelched his impulse to comment.

"The bad news is, I still have to insist on the pay cut. The numbers just don't add up otherwise. You know what I always say: 'If it ain't in the cards, you can't play the hand.' The good news is, we can probably make this cut only once, if—and only if—we can put some teeth into our policies regarding scheduling, cancellations, and waiting times.

"There are a couple of really bad apples in the barrel, Joshua. You know who they are. They're costing us money and morale. You promised me you'd pull the Board into line on that one."

Joshua focused on placidly sipping his coffee. He wasn't about to swallow this hook today, especially after the barbs he'd already taken at the board meeting.

"I'll get to that later if we have time," Joshua said, putting his cup down. "Let me get this clear. Are you telling me we have absolutely no choice but to implement the cuts on payroll and the 401 retirement contribution? There's nothing you can do?"

Damien locked his eyes on Joshua's and spoke through clenched teeth. "Come on, Joshua. We've been over this before. If we freeze the staff's raises again this year, we'll virtually lay the red carpet for a union takeover. I've butchered the staff training and development budget. And," he paused and flicked an extended finger toward Joshua, "without touching the doctors' professional leave, I might add."

Joshua sat silently. His stoic appearance made Damien feel as if he were out on the limb by himself. He rose to his feet, holding out his hands and shaking his head in genuine frustration. "You make it sound like this is my fault. You say, 'Is there nothing you can do?' as if I'm the one always asking for the biggest and best piece of equipment. As if I'm the one who cancels patients left and right, so I can go play golf. The board members tell me I've got the tail wagging the dog. Well, it seems to me as if a lot of your buddies treat the staff around here like they were dogs. If one of my people treated another staff member the way some of those doctors do, it would be cause for immediate dismissal!"

Joshua held up his hand. "Damien, cool down. What I really mean is 'Is there anything we can do?' You're not the only one taking heat these days." He looked intently at Damien, hoping for some sign whether or not he was aware of what had gone on at the board meeting.

"So I heard." Damien flexed his hair-covered fingers and slid back into his desk chair. "You know, I could've armed you with an updated list of bullet points if you had told me about it beforehand."

Thank God. Damien didn't know about the memo. Or, if he did, Damien was a better poker player than Joshua had ever given him credit for. "They needed to vent their spleens. They want another meeting next week. Can you get me those bullets by the end of the day Monday?"

111

"Another closed meeting?" Damien's voice revealed his true feelings even as he leaned back in his chair.

"I don't like them any better than you do. You know that. But there's no point in adding fuel to the fire by objecting to it."

Joshua paused. Would the word "fire" elicit any reaction from Damien? When it didn't, Joshua moved forward cautiously. "Besides, I've got a few ideas that may help them bite the bullet."

Leaning forward, Damien looked Joshua straight in the eyes. "Get off it, Joshua. I know we've not always been on the same side of the fence, but don't tease me like one of your trout. If you don't want to tell me what you have in mind, just say so. Don't make me ask."

"Fair enough. You've certainly heard about my lunch with Dr. Moerae King. She's an organizational psychologist that Jane ran into. I'm considering recommending her consulting services to the board."

"A real looker, so I heard. But what does she know about financial stuff?"

Joshua curled his fingers into an O. "Nothing directly—as far as I can tell. That's not her thing. But she's working for some really big outfits—"

Damien interrupted, "Which means she ain't cheap."

Joshua shook his head. Good old predictable Damien. He continued, "We aren't the only ones getting bounced around these days. I think—I hope—that the financial heat we're experiencing is nothing more what she would call normal growing pains. Anyway, she's developing a proposal for diagnosing whatever it is that ails our organizational culture. I'll arrange for you two to meet soon."

Joshua smiled inwardly at the deep sigh that escaped Damien's lips. You got it. There's no percentage in fighting me on this one.

"As long as I don't get blamed for her fees! Anything else on your agenda?" Damien asked swiveling back and forth.

The timing was not quite right to tell Damien this now, but he felt compelled to. "Just one more thing. We lost a patient this morning: Mrs. Susan Wong. Take a look at her bill and let me know if there's anything we can do to keep it to a bare minimum. The family has coverage but the deductible will hit them pretty hard."

Warning bells went off in Damien's mind. His frown made his face look like a photograph from a house of mirrors. "Is she shark bait?"

"I seriously doubt it. We had a good relationship, but I've got Ross doing an autopsy this morning. I'll let you know what he finds. She was just a nice lady." He straightened up and changed his tone. "Let me know when you get those bullets together."

Damien turned back to his computer. "I'll get on it right now."

Damien Rees was all business, and when it came to business, the bottom line was all that really mattered. Even before Joshua was out the door, Damien was typing a special password into his computer. As the screen blinked, a list of patient names stared back at him. He invoked the search command and tapped out the patient's name, SUSAN WONG.

As the computer raced through millions of bytes of information, Damien reflected on the simple little game he had discovered when his first real love, John, had contracted AIDS.

An insurance company approached them with a proposition that would help John and Damien handle the burden of their astronomically mounting medical expenses. "Viatical settlements" the company called them. Damien was too proud to ask what it meant, but he later found it in the dictionary. The term was from the Latin viaticum, meaning "provisions for a journey."

The company, Care Inc., would advance them fifty percent of John's half-million-dollar life insurance policy immediately, giving John and Damien the opportunity to fulfill some of their fondest dreams. All John had to do was reassign the policy, naming Care Inc. the prime beneficiary upon his death.

Care Inc. didn't have to wait very long for a very handsome return on its investment. One day while Damien was out of town, John wandered out of their apartment in a drugged stupor and ended up at Cook County Hospital—in the AIDS ward with no bars or screens on its tenth-floor windows. Damien swallowed back a lump rising in his throat as he recalled the long, panic-filled day it took to find what was left of John after he'd jumped out of that hospital window.

The irony of it all! John had willed the remaining advance money to Damien. And Damien used it to start his nursing home business. Damien—at his opportunistic best—then struck a deal with Care, Inc. to sell them records of patients who were good prospects for similar insurance advances. The nursing home was fertile ground for Care, Inc., so Damien was able to use this additional capital to grow his company. And it was this rapid growth that had attracted Joshua to Damien and convinced Joshua to hire him.

Now he had a much larger, more fertile database to prospect. Dipping into C.C.A.'s patient records was a piece of cake for Damien. While his high school friends were out wasting their time chasing girls, Damien had spent all of his time alone learning the intricacies of computers. Hacking around in even sophisticated systems was second nature to him now. He knew this system inside-out, for he had led the IT committee in selecting it. And by not having to bring in an outside computer consultant, he saved them a pretty bundle doing so. They had no reason to complain—nor to suspect anything.

Then to make it even sweeter, he managed to get Paul Blake to feed him the inside scoop about patients' medical prognoses. What a perfect coup!

His monitor blinked Susan Wong's name. She was one of "his." She had accepted Care, Inc.'s offer to advance her $100,000 against her policy's $200,000 face value.

No big deal. But then again, a fifteen percent cut, split fifty-fifty, was a damn good return on investment for the time involved. "If it ain't in the cards, you can't play the hand," Damien whispered. He leaned back and patted his firm flat belly, deeply satisfied with himself. The doctors' decks would be ten percent smaller this year, but, he noted with pride, his would be more than full. He put his mind to getting Joshua the bullets he would need.

❧

Joshua passed by Mary's desk. "Has Ross come by?"

"He just arrived a few minutes ago. He's in your office. How did it go?"

"The internal bleeding has stopped for now," Joshua said as he slammed his door behind him.

Ross Benson slouched his tall, lanky frame on Joshua's couch. He had a pathology journal in one hand and a Diet Coke in the other.

Joshua chuckled. "With all the rusty-pipe organs you've seen in your day, I'm surprised you can put that stuff into your stomach."

Ross smiled back, but wouldn't look directly at Joshua. He hoisted the can in a mock toast and said, "To each his own poison, as they say."

Joshua shrugged his shoulders and dropped heavily into his leather chair. He eyed Ross with apprehension and admiration. Ross had been at his side through many an important battle inside C.C.A. He had initiated the Impaired Physicians Committee and regular mortality conferences. While Joshua chaired those meetings, Ross never failed to sit at his right hand and support him through the sometimes painful proceedings.

Ross's trained eye and years of experience could ultimately determine whether or not an entire career went down the tubes. Sure, the doctors on the hot seat might be able to get a job somewhere else, but their lives and those of their families would never be the same. A million successes were never enough to cancel out one avoidable mistake.

The unpredictability of practicing medicine guaranteed that Ross himself had taken his turn in the hot seat more than once, most recently in a case involving a suspected bone cancer. Lay people thought pathology was merely a matter of looking at a slide and a neon light would flash "malignant" or "benign." Were that the case, a fourteen-year-old girl might not have lost an arm unnecessarily a few months before. But if Ross's diagnosis had been wrong, and they didn't amputated soon enough, the girl might never have celebrated her sixteenth birthday. Medicine could be a cruel and fickle business.

Wondering if it were-his turn on the seat, Joshua faced Ross and took a deep breath. "Yesterday went smooth as silk. No complications. Her heart was pumping up a storm."

Thank God, Ross wasn't sadistic by nature. He could easily use Joshua's anxiety as an opportunity to get even for the scene at the board meeting.

"She just got tired, Joshua. Her engine had run its last mile. There was absolutely nothing you or anyone else could've done."

Death from natural causes was the most common end to most lives. Yet, to an overwhelming majority of physicians totally committed to doing their best, it was one of the hardest things to write down on a death certificate. It simply meant they could do nothing.

Joshua rose, exhaled deeply and sat down on the couch next to Ross. "Thanks, Ross. I'm really grateful you happened to be in today."

"You're welcome," Ross said. For an instant, the two men looked at one another peacefully.

Joshua broke the silence. "Look, Ross, I'm sorry for the accusation I made about you at the meeting. I was really pissed at being blindsided by that memo."

Ross said nothing. His avocado green eyes never wavered from Joshua's gaze.

Joshua cleared his throat. "I didn't want to then and don't want to now believe that you'd be the instigator of an attempt at a bloodless coup. The stress just got to me. I'm sorry."

"Bloodless coup?" Ross repeated. "In this business, isn't that an oxymoron?" Both laughed. "I share many of their concerns, Joshua, but I tried to talk them out of presenting you with a fait accompli. Once the fire got roaring, it was impossible to stop."

Joshua remembered his conversation with Peter earlier in the morning. It seemed ages ago. He wanted to test the idea with Ross. "Peter came up with an idea this morning that may just be the counter-fire we need to prevent this from burning out of control. Have you got a few extra minutes now?"

Five minutes later, the two longtime friends shook hands, of one mind. Two-thirds of the Financial Review Committee was in place.

They walked out of the office and Joshua stopped in front of Mary's desk. "Go home already, will you? But before you go, would you please call Ruth and tell her I'm on my way?"

———

She nodded.

"I'm thinking about going fishing tomorrow," he said to Ross as they started walking.

"I doubt it," Mary called out to him. "There's a storm blowing in off the lake."

"Be sure to tell Ruth that, too. It'll make her day. She'll have to put up with me the entire weekend. See you Monday."

Eight

Stretching in her hotel bed, Moerae luxuriated in a windfall of unexpected time on a Saturday morning. She'd been scheduled to give a speech to the Omaha Rotary Club, but had gotten an apologetic call at 7 a.m. to inform her the president of the club had passed away suddenly during the night. She felt bad about the death. It was a hell of a reason to cancel a gathering, but she thanked the heavens for some precious hours to herself.

Freed from other obligations, her mind floated freely from idea to idea searching for the perfect way to frame the proposal she'd promised Joshua. She was reasonably sure that Joshua was nearly sold on the idea of bringing her in, but how could she best phrase the proposal for Joshua to sell it to his board?

The white sheets tightened around her exquisite form as she rolled toward the nightstand. Moerae firmly believed that the greatest testament ever written to the principles of total quality management was not to be found on the shelves of business school libraries, but rather, in the book found in the drawer next to every hotel bed in the country. She fished the Bible out of her bedside table and fingered the false leather cover for a moment before thumbing through the pages with practiced ease to find the commandment she most loved: *Do unto others as you would have them do unto you.*

So simple, and yet how difficult to remember. Did the creators of the now-coveted Baldridge Award for Quality ever reach for the grace of this wisdom, Christian or not? Most of her professional colleagues seemed to waste everyone's time and effort by complicating the simple and obvious truths in life. Did they think their clients wouldn't pay for simplicity? In many instances, she noted cynically, they were probably right.

Moerae had once written for one of her professional journals a little piece called "Making Believe: The Game of Organizational Development." She scripted it as a Greek tragedy. While the rhetoric between consultant and client was dramatized onstage, the chorus recited what was really going on as an aside:

"You'll make believe you don't know what needs to be done to solve the problem," the consultant advises. "Then you can hire me at a very high fee, because the problem is so difficult that it has defied your ability to solve it. I will arrive and, with great empathy, confirm that the problem is indeed very serious, and that a very long and protracted therapy is needed to heal the illness. To reinforce this charade, you will ask me to give you a very detailed list of proposals and recommendations that affirms how terribly complicated the problem is, written in mystical consultant language so filled with jargon it will be incomprehensible to the layman. In fact, we will emphasize at the outset that we do not even know what the problem is. Together, we will collude in denying that the solution is actually quite simple."

Moerae felt the sting of her own conscience as she sat up against three plumped pillows and gazed at the light filtering through the gauzy curtains. Easy to talk about *Truth*, she thought, harder to actually live it. How many years had she hidden in the closet? The truth was uncomplicated. She loved women. But in order to experience the freeing power of this truth, she first had to admit that she'd imprisoned herself behind the walls of denial. The longer she fed her own lies, the stronger they became. And the stronger they grew, the more she had to struggle to speak her heart out loud.

A knock at the door snapped her head. "Room service, Dr. King," a voice called out.

She'd forgotten about ordering breakfast the night before. "Hang on a second," she shouted back, pulling on her robe. "I'll be right with you."

When she opened the door and a young woman stood leaning slightly sideways under the weight of a heavily laden tray, Moerae felt a shudder ripple through her spine as if she were looking into a mirror that distorted time instead of shape.

The young woman shifted her weight from one foot to the other. "Excuse me, ma'am, but can you tell me where you'd like me to put this?"

"Oh, of course. I'm sorry. Please put it here," Moerae pointed toward the coffee table. The woman entered the room briskly, swinging the tray smoothly down onto the table in a practiced movement, and presented it squarely to face Moerae when she sat down. "You've come a long way, baby," Moerae uttered under her breath.

"Pardon?" the younger woman asked.

"Oh, excuse me. I was just reminding myself of something," Moerae said, smiling broadly. "I used to work part-time as a room service waitress when I was going to college. Seeing you standing there brought back memories."

The young woman leaned over the table and poured Moerae a cup of coffee. "I hope to go to college some day, ma'am. Right now I'm just trying to help my mama and take care of my baby."

The girl sounded exhausted underneath her cheerful facade. Moerae reached into her purse for a tip, knowing that the cash would go directly into the girl's pocket, instead of into a pool to be shared with everyone else.

121

"Thank you, ma'am. Just put the tray outside the door when you're finished and I'll come and fetch it."

"Good luck getting to college," she said, knowing full well that the girl's odds were flimsy at best. Moerae dialed the front desk and, in a matter of moments, thanks to a truly service-oriented concierge, got a late check out, a Do Not Disturb lock on her phone, and an assurance a cab would be waiting when she needed it.

Moerae reached for the cup of coffee. "That's better," she said, licking her lips. The decaf was just as she liked. The hotel's management kept careful track of their customers' likes and dislikes. Too bad the health care organizations she worked with couldn't do as good a job of making people feel at home.

Biting into a muffin, Moerae scanned the front page of the newspaper. Her eyes darted back and forth between the headlines until the words and images on the page rose up and dissolved like the shifting shapes in a kaleidoscope. She admitted to herself she had no stomach for the world's bad news this morning, and tossed the paper aside.

She reached for the speech she'd prepared for the Rotarians. She was confident that the professional and business people based in and around Omaha would be very familiar with scriptures. So the thrust of her speech centered on an imaginary annual report made to the stockholders of Earth, Inc. She diligently chose buzzwords that might be both familiar and comfortable to business people. Mission, authority, responsibility, policies, procedures. Moerae munched mechanically on the remains of her English muffin as she reviewed her manuscript.

As we approach the start of our third millennium, I feel the need to take stock of Earth, Inc.'s business history and future. Our fundamental mission, albeit under increasingly severe threat and attack, is unchanged. That mission is to become an even more loving, beautiful and creative planet, a perfect reflection of my cosmic Being. Earth, fire, water, and air remain the essential elements needed to support our business. How dare we forget that these elements are finite, both in supply and quality, and they are susceptible to abuse.

Moerae picked up a croissant and stopped reading to spread a generous spoonful of peach jam on it. Why can't we remember these simple truths? In this business called "Life" we are all CEOs responsible for our choices and their consequences. Unless we regularly take stock of our actions and values—and rid ourselves of those that fail to support our mission of becoming loving, caring people—we will only continue to slide into moral, spiritual and emotional bankruptcy. The evidence is in our faces every day, in the papers, on the TV and in our corporate boardrooms. We're surrounded by the ruin and destruction of abusive power mongers, hell-bent on feeding their own ravenous appetites.

She stepped into the bathroom, her mind still racing. The history of executives abusing power—corporate, political and military—unfolded like a perverse tapestry in her imagination. Male-dominated leadership has for centuries promulgated a conqueror-oppressor model. And once total dominance is achieved, the dominator no longer has to live by his own rules.

Moerae stared in the mirror over the porcelain sink while she washed her hands. Women were beginning to gain the recognition they deserved in the world of management, but it was a slow invasion of this historical "boys' club." Certainly, she thought, the day will come when the masculine and feminine sides of human nature could function as equals. But in the meantime, the power dynamics in existing world hierarchies mostly reflected an unconscious preoccupation with the comparative control over "all things great and small."

What she most wanted to convey to the board members of C.C.A. was that spiritual bankruptcy is indeed the greatest threat to its survival. But a room full of men—doctors who fancied themselves as men of science—wouldn't easily sit still for talk about "spiritual" issues. She would have to construct her terms very carefully, or she'd be laughed out of the boardroom.

Moerae bent over the coffee table to pick up the tray and leave it outside the door, but she thought twice and stopped. She remembered her friend from room service and decided to leave the tray where it was, hoping that the young waiter's shift would be over before she checked out. This simple act of compassion revealed Moerae's heart as she thought out loud, "One less load for her to have to pick up and carry alone."

Nine

As he entered the board meeting, Joshua felt lighter than he had a week ago. Body less tense. Blood not boiling. Was it the upper he'd popped with his coffee? No, he had reason for cautious optimism. Roger Rosen had enthusiastically agreed to join with Peter and Ross to form an internal finance review committee. When the word had leaked out, several of Joshua's colleagues had acknowledged him with a nod when they passed him in the halls during the past few days. This had lifted his spirits considerably, even in the face of the discontented buzz still dominating the doctors' dining room.

In addition, he'd been pleasantly surprised that Moerae had given him her proposal early. Her insights made the hair on the back of his neck stand up, as if she'd been sitting at his side during recent conversations. Although many of the challenges she listed probably weren't specific to C.C.A., her prognosis was uncannily accurate.

The most pertinent points were enough to justify hiring her. A steep decline in morale stood out, clearly reflected in the increasing staff turnover. It obviously affected more than the rank and file, too. It had become almost unbearably difficult to attract and hold high earners among the physicians; and that only increased delays in patient access. This was an immediate deterioration of their ability to provide service, and how else was their business defined?

But staring at him in black and white for him—and the board—to see, the clearest evidence of C.C.A.'s disease was the financial one. It showed the organization living ever closer to the edge of the credit vortex, which could eventually suck the whole operation down the drain. C.C.A.'s increasing debt load was causing lines of credit to tighten up, while at the same time the pinched cash flow brought very heavy pressure to borrow more—just to cover operations, let alone needed expansion.

Behind the symptoms, though, Moerae's report revealed her conviction that Joshua had never viewed C.C.A. as a living, breathing organism. It had always seemed somehow separate from the people in it. Yet Moerae had led him to understand that without people, the concept of an organization made no sense.

But most haunting was her personal cover letter to him. He couldn't shake the evocative biblical references she'd made, in particular one cited from Mishnah, Sanhedrin 4:5:

"Therefore was one single man created first, Adam, to teach you that if anyone destroys a single soul from the children of man, Scripture charges him as though he had destroyed a whole universe and whoever rescues a single soul from the children of man, Scripture credits him as if he had saved a whole universe."

What was it about this passage that disturbed him so? It stirred something, presented a challenge he couldn't quite articulate. He resolved to speak with Moerae about it at the first opportunity.

Joshua slid into his chair at the head of the table and called the meeting to order. "The sooner we get started, the sooner we can all go home," he began.

Paul Blake scowled and glanced pointedly at Mary Howard. "I thought we'd agreed that this would be a closed meeting."

"I'm sorry, Paul. I'll explain Mary's presence," Joshua began. What luck that the ringleader of the star chamber group had identified himself so early in the meeting instead of leaving the job to one of his pawns. "Damien promised to give us some up-to-date figures for the meeting. They've just arrived and Mary is still putting together the details for me. I hope this meets with your approval?" He raised an eyebrow at Paul.

"Uh, no problem." Paul smiled weakly, settling back into his chair. "I just wanted to make sure we were all in agreement that Damien wouldn't be here today."

Joshua looked away from Paul, but addressed his next remark to him. "As you can all appreciate, when I met with Damien, I made it clear that the board wished to continue their discussions in private. He didn't like that." He glared at Scott MacDonald. "But since the news of our last meeting came as no surprise to him, he didn't make a big deal out of it."

Scott's dimpled lower jaw dropped open and his catcher's mitt hand jerked reflexively. Before he could start mewling, Joshua said, "Relax, Scott. I'm not interested in laying the blame on anyone. I just wanted you all to understand that at the same time I would not invite Damien to this meeting, I had no intention of hiding it from him. Nor is there any way I can legislate what any of you do with the facts that result from our discussions today."

The drug in his veins rushed with a cool heat and his brain kept pace with it, never missing a beat. Joshua saved this old trout fishing trick for very important occasions so as not to lessen its effect. He'd cast his hook a few times in a different section of the pool, well away from the fish he wanted to snag, lulling the fellow into a false sense of security. Targeting Scott might flush out bigger game lurking in the shadows.

"Let's not beat around the bush, gentlemen. Unless Damien has uncovered some dramatically new information in the past couple of days, the bottom line is that we have absolutely no choice but to take a ten percent cut in pay across the board this year." Joshua looked toward Mary.

She shrugged as she passed him the papers.

Scott piped up, his voice squeaking. "What about the 401(k) retirement contributions? Are we going to lose those too?"

"You announcing your retirement, Scott?" Joshua couldn't help himself.

Scott's face flushed to match his red suspenders. "That's not funny, Joshua."

"No, it's not," Joshua said. "I apologize. Give me a minute. I just got these, as I said." He put his reading glasses on, lowered his head and began shuffling through the papers, buying a few seconds to formulate his response. "Why don't you guys fill me in on your discussions after last week's meeting while I scan these?" he said without looking up.

"We just went out for a drink to unwind," Paul said.

Joshua forced a cough to keep his felicity at bay. "These are very serious times," he said, still keeping his head down as if he hadn't noticed Paul's gaffe. "I assume you've all been as concerned as I have with our situation. I could really use the benefit of everyone's thoughts and discussions," he added.

Paul's deeply set smoky eyes narrowed into slits, balefully staring at Joshua. Joshua had conned him into sticking the hook into himself. His bony hands gripped the arms of his chair with enough force to turn his knuckles white. Grinding his teeth, his pointed jaw jutted out as if inviting a blow.

"Are you all right?" Joshua asked.

Paul snarled, "What do you mean?"

"You really ought to sign up for a complete physical, Paul. I'm worried about you. Your face is as red as your Porsche." Joshua pasted on a concerned frown.

"If it helps any, the scuttlebutt around town is that everyone else is in much worse shape than we are," Jane Sherwood began, an appeasing smile on her innocent face.

The two men turned to her reluctantly.

"The senior executives of Family Health are being sued for taking a pay increase while denying a terminally ill patient access to a very expensive procedure," she continued. "The patient subsequently died. Mount Sinai is about to lose their entire cardiology department en masse. Saint Elizabeth's billing system is so screwed up that the bank is about to squeeze down on their line of credit. And word is that Big Blue is going to take over managing them on a day-to-day basis."

Peter jumped in. "Nice guys, those bankers. They'll lend you all the money you want when you don't need it. But as soon as they see any blood, they pinch down on your IV and cut back on your transfusions. What our friendly shark," Peter continued, smiling at Jane, "is trying to hammer through our thick heads is that there's no cause for panic. We're a long way from having our absentee third-party landlords moving in with us."

"Easy for you to say! You don't have to work for a living like some of us!" Scott whined, right on cue. "We all know you're our resident Wall Street guru."

Peter grinned. "Thank you very much for the vote of confidence."

Ross tapped his manicured willowy fingers on the table. "If you'll hold your horses a minute, Scott, Joshua has an idea as to how we might be able to use Peter's financial wizardry to our advantage."

"Why don't you and Peter and Roger fill them in?" Joshua asked, waving them on. "There may be a glimmer of hope in this mess of paper and I need a few more minutes to check it out. I don't want to raise any false hopes, but we may be able to salvage a portion of the 401(k) monies."

Everyone, including Joshua, looked up in surprise as Roger Rosen stood. It was quite uncharacteristic for Roger to be so forward.

"If I might?" Roger asked.

Peter and Ross both nodded.

In a measured voice, Roger carefully began. "Look, we're just like all the other doctors in this place. We can barely keep up on our own specialties. I'm a heart surgeon, not an accountant, and what I don't understand makes me suspicious. I just want to do what I was trained to do. What I love to do. I love seeing the look on a patient's face when they wake up and see a familiar, loved one's face smiling back at them instead of St. Peter's. That's what I'm here for, and I believe that's what most of us are here for."

Joshua felt Roger's eyes on him and he looked up from the papers. Those ebony eyes were boring into him. Roger continued with rising passion in his voice, "I've got to tell you, Joshua, when you first asked me to join with Peter and Ross on a special Finance Review Committee, I was suspicious as all hell! I don't know squat about finance, and Peter isn't exactly a neutral member of this board!"

"If I'd wanted a neutral finance audit, I would've gone outside the board," Joshua retorted. "You guys don't trust Damien because he isn't a doctor. You don't seem to have much more faith in me, for that matter. Is there anything that will satisfy you guys?"

Roger glared at Joshua. "I'd like to finish, if you could just hold your temper for a minute."

Joshua took off his glasses, rubbed his temples and sighed heavily. "I'm sorry, Roger. But, you know, I'm just a surgeon too. And, I'm not getting a lot of time to do what I love these days, plus I'm catching more heat as well. I apologize, but this is a pretty thankless position sometimes. Everything I do seems to piss off somebody in this group!"

Everyone sat in stunned silent stillness. The depth of his feelings caught even Joshua by surprise. His pulse pounded in his ears. The babies he was taking were supposed to keep such vulnerability under control.

Roger rubbed his mustache and broke the awkward tension. "I almost decided to turn down Joshua's request, but I thought I'd check with Ross first. When he told me that Peter was to be given a completely free rein and that we wouldn't be obligated to give preliminary feedback to Joshua, I was all for it." Roger turned to his chief. "That's not because I don't trust you, Joshua. The fact that you'd give us absolutely freedom in these matters, trusting us to give all the information we've gathered to the group first, only reaffirms my faith in you."

"I thank you for that," Joshua said, a slight catch in his voice. He was embarrassed by his outburst, but Roger's reassurance of loyalty simultaneously soothed him. Jesus, how deeply fear had embedded itself throughout the entire structure of C.C.A. And he was no more immune to its effects than anyone else in the room.

Joshua cleared his throat and looked down at his papers to collect himself before addressing his council. "The work of this committee is absolutely vital. If the doctors lose all faith and trust, they will stampede, and that kind of internal bleeding could really put us over the edge. The only way we can succeed is to put forward our most wholehearted cooperation. I expect each and every one of us to be fully available to support the committee in any way they need us."

He glanced over at Mary. "Nothing takes priority on my calendar."

She nodded.

"Now, if you're ready, gentlemen, I may have some good news about the retirement issue. It looks as if we may be able to cover at least a part of the amount required if—and it's a *big* IF—

we can plug up some of the most obvious, chronic leaks in our own systems."

Paul made no effort to disguise his disdain. "Like what?"

"For one, some of our colleagues are not meeting their appointment schedules. I've noticed a strange coincidence: Cancellations increase on unusually sunny afternoons when conditions are perfect for golf. For another thing, many of us are not keeping our charts up to date. I'm sorry to say that I'm one of the worst offenders in this regard."

"We've been over these issues before, Joshua. What's going to be different this time?" Paul asked. Paul's vitriolic riposte left him on his back foot, fists clenched, cocked in readiness for a brawl.

"Given the way information travels through this place, I'm sure you're all aware that I had lunch with an organizational consultant last week," Joshua stated calmly.

"I don't want some time-and-motion expert hanging over my shoulder!" Scott Macdonald blurted.

Peter leered, "*You* obviously didn't see her, Scott!" The men burst into laughter. Scott looked like a lost puppy. Peter cupped both his hands to his chest. Scott's bug eyes opened wide and his tongue crossed his chunky lips.

Jane Sherwood smiled, but grimly. "I might add that her brains are even more impressive than her boobs, and she has worked with some of the largest health care organizations in the country."

"Excuse our behavior, Jane, we mean no disrespect," Joshua said. He pushed a manila folder toward the center of the table. "Dr. Moerae King has responded with enthusiasm and remarkable speed to our dilemma, for which I'm grateful. You're all welcome to read her full proposal. In fact, I encourage you to do so. She'll be making a preliminary diagnosis to see if she can help us address exactly the kind of questions you raised, Paul.

What's wrong with us? We seem to rehash certain important issues time and again without ever resolving them. Why has personnel turnover grown to average almost twenty percent a year? Why do physician salaries and benefits continue to decrease as a percentage of collected dollars?

"She'll be conducting interviews in the next week or so." Turning to Mary, he continued, "Mary will call to schedule time with each of you. I've asked Dr. King to have a preliminary report delivered to us at the opening session of our long planning retreat in two weeks."

Mary quickly thumbed through her notes. "Opening session on June 29, after cocktails and dinner at the Country Club. Scheduled to start at five-thirty sharp."

"What's she going to cost?" Paul asked.

"Less-than you charge to put some people to sleep. And I guarantee you that she won't do that to you." Joshua slid the manila envelope across the polished tabletop.

Paul sneered as he reached to snatch the folder.

"I'll ask Damien to work up some more spreadsheets on the issues we've discussed today." Joshua rose, tapping the sheaf of papers on the desk. He took several deep breaths, deliberately pacing himself as he looked around the table. "I'll ask him to present a specific set of recommendations to us ... at our next regularly scheduled board meeting."

Ten

Damien Rees was the first interview Moerae arranged on her schedule. At his suggestion, it began with her sitting in on one of his regular staff meetings.

The small meeting room adjoined Damien's office. The large table looked like a slab of highly polished obsidian. Reflected in its mirror-like surface were neatly arranged stacks of paper, set at regular intervals in front of each chair. Next to each stack lay three newly sharpened pencils of exactly the same length, aligned in military precision. No erasers, Moerae noted. Damien would not anticipate mistakes. His staff would get it right, and get it right the first time.

Damien was businesslike but cordial to her. He introduced her to the staff as a corporate psychologist who'd been invited in to help "shrink the size of the doctors' egos," which excited a polite ripple of amusement around the table.

Moerae declined his offer of the seat next to him. "I prefer to sit with the Indians. That way, I can keep an eye on the chief."

Right off the bat, the staff took their cues from Damien. Because he demonstrated no anxiety at her presence, neither did anyone else. No self-conscious shrinking into silence or stiffening. Within minutes, Moerae felt herself fitting seamlessly into the group.

This spoke well of Damien. As interested in control as he seemed to be, he got results. A polished performer, the man was cunning and powerful. He certainly could not have survived this long in his position at C.C.A. without these qualities. And how easily these high-ranking members of his team seemed to accept the rigor of his expectations. Damien was an administrative satrap of a certain stripe.

Notably, all those present were clearly on their best behavior. The code of conduct to which each adhered with strict attention was no less rigid because it was invisible. Moerae had questioned Mary Howard and learned that Damien's methods could be harsh. Random reprimands, public humiliation, subtle shifts in responsibility were periodically visited on staff who broke out of line. Anyone who had ever offended Damien's sensibilities did so only once.

The meeting was productive and quick, as Damien conducted business in a crisp, orderly manner. Much of their work involved managing their other bosses, the doctors, and in this challenge they were all united.

Damien didn't break form until he and Moerae had retired to his private office. "So what did you think of the meeting, Dr. King?"

"It was one of the most orderly and productive meetings I've observed in a long while. I'm very impressed with your ability to stay focused on the agenda."

Damien ducked his head to hide his reddening cheeks. She was happy to see he responded to sincere praise, but his need to cover it up amused her. A little boy who wanted to be noticed for his achievements and would respond to encouragement lived inside that crusty exterior.

Damien nodded gracefully. "Thank you, Dr. King. Coming from someone with your credentials and experience, I take that as a real compliment. I know my staff will appreciate hearing that as well, if you have no objection to my passing it on." He glanced toward the pot on the spotless table. "Are you coffeed out, or would you like another cup?"

"No, thank you."

Damien sat at his desk, leaving her to decide where to sit. She chose the finely-brocaded armchair beside the desk instead of the hardback directly in front of him. More intimate.

She threw her first question in the hopes of getting an unrehearsed reaction from Damien. "Do any of the doctors ever attend your staff meetings?"

Damien's scarred jaw stiffened involuntarily, and when he spoke his voice was steely. "Except for Joshua, I mean Dr. Caliban," he quickly corrected, "we don't get many doctors visiting us in administration. And when they do, you'd think we were the blood bank. Do you mind if I ask why you wanted to know?"

As she suspected. The little boy had been wounded. Damien's pride, which she intuited was enormous, had turned to bitterness. The physicians had either failed to recognize his hardearned achievements or, worse, belittled them. She had to find out how seriously the damage had eroded his better nature.

She tilted her head and began slowly, "What I have noticed in many instances in the health care field is that the we-they dynamics characterizing the relationships between physicians and non-physicians and between management and staff blinds all of us to the commonality of our purpose. The result of these dysfunctional relationships is that *dis*-ease sets in and works like a cancer, spreading throughout the entire organism until it ultimately affects the patients—and I cannot exaggerate this enough—sometimes fatally. Does this reflect your observations of what's happening in C.C.A.?"

Damien's bushy brows curled inward, his rounded lips pursed. "Come, come, Dr. King. That's a bit dramatic, isn't it?

Doctors are busy people. Their job is to treat patients. We don't want them wasting their time hanging around administration."

Moerae raised an eyebrow. Could Damien hear the condescending tone of his own voice? She'd learned what she needed. Damien was as much in denial of other people's truths as anyone else here.

"My mother always told me I should have been an actress," she said, chuckling. "I'm sure Dr. Caliban must have told you that I see organizations as living beings. So tell me a little bit about the patient from your point of view. How healthy an organism is C.C.A.?"

The rest of their conversation was cordial and relaxed. Damien assured her again and again that C.C.A. had its moods, its ups and downs, aches and pains, just like any other business, but was fundamentally sound.

"So, would it be fair to say that based on your view of C.C.A. there's no need for any outside consultation?"

Damien shifted nervously and stated flatly, "Dr Caliban doesn't tell me how to manage my administrative staff, Dr. King, and I wouldn't presume to tell him how to manage the doctors."

"Dr. Caliban was very open about the problems you're having with the doctors." She paused for effect. "He did, however, promise me I would have free rein to look at the entire organization."

"Absolutely. Just let me know who within my area you want to see and I'll make certain you get their full cooperation. We all have room to improve," Damien said.

In spite of his pinching his hairy nostrils as he spoke, the turned down corner of Damien's round lips belied his true attitude even as he assured her of full cooperation. Its significance did not escape Moerae's experienced eyes.

"Thank you," was all she said.

Damien returned her smile and opened his hands. "I'm sure you know how difficult it can be, being a prophet in your own land. The doctors don't hear my words when I speak. Anything you can do to help my people get the recognition they deserve from the doctors will be greatly appreciated."

She couldn't have said it better herself. She flashed her most brilliant smile and stood up, reaching across the corner of his desk to shake his hand. "I'll do my best. You've been most helpful." She started toward the door as she added, "I have another appointment this morning that I need to get to."

A quiet sigh of relief escaped Damien's lips as he hurried to walk her out. "I enjoyed talking with you. Please don't hesitate to ask for any help we might be able to provide."

In Damien's outer office, a tall, lanky, sallow-faced doctor thumbing through a magazine waited to see Damien. Moerae noticed Damien's face light up, so she concluded this visiting M.D. wasn't there "to get blood"—at least not from Damien. She wished she could read the name plate on the man's white coat. His bent head also prevented her from seeing his eyes, but most likely they'd one day be introduced. And she sensed it wasn't a meeting she looked forward to.

"Dr. Albert's office is just across the courtyard on the third floor of the main building," Damien said casually as he skillfully guided her toward the door.

Moerae felt a dampness in her palms. She'd been very careful not to mention anything about her next appointment. Damien's command of the information flow within C.C.A. was very thorough, as with every other system he controlled. The fact that he knew her itinerary wasn't a big deal. What caught her attention was the chilled correctness of his voice. Damien *expected* to be aware of these kinds of details.

"Thanks," she said.

As the outer door closed, Moerae saw Damien put his hand on his visitor's thin bony shoulder out of the corner of her eye.

❧

As Damien was ushering his visitor out of his office, Paul Blake had purposefully avoided any eye contact with her. He had already known who was behind Damien's closed door, thanks to his secretary. Dr. Blake prided himself on getting women to open up to him and she had offered little resistance to his cajoling questions. "Oh, you mean Dr. King," had come rolling off her lips. Immediately Paul noticed her self-conscious expression, so he assured her he wouldn't tell Damien of her slip of the tongue because he knew it could cost her a severe reprimand.

"Come on in. Sorry I'm a bit late," Damien said.

Paul stiffened at Damien's touch of his shoulder. Being at the top of an uneven table was the best playing field, and the way to assure that position was to keep your cards hidden while getting others to show theirs'. He had told Damien many times not to get physical with him in public. The less people at C.C.A. knew about him, the better.

"No problem. Gave me a chance to get to know your secretary better," he said, making sure Damien saw the wink he gave her.

"Make sure we're not interrupted. Dr. Blake and I have some important matters to discuss," Damien called back as he closed his office door.

"What the hell are you doing kissing up to my secretary?" Damien said through clenched teeth.

Paul gave him a quick hug and then broke before Damien could respond. "Just reminding you to keep your hands to yourself in public. Don't get your balls in an uproar. We've got more important matters to discuss."

Damien sighed and finally nodded. "This broad is someone not to be taken lightly."

Paul sat on Damien's couch and patted the cushion next to him. Controlling how the conversation went would be easier if he let Damien have some physical contact. "So fill me in."

"I'll tell you right off that unless she's bullshitting me, she's got Joshua in the palm of her hand."

Paul leaned forward and waved his long arm in a dismissive gesture. "Data! Data! Not editorial interpretations."

"Well, for example, she stressed that Joshua had assured her free rein, and I quote, 'to the entire organization.'"

Rather than be concerned about Damien's example, Paul felt relieved. What was it that the disguised bad wolf had said to little Red Riding Hood when she commented on his big eyes—something about "the easier to see you with?"

"Not to worry. The more visible she is, the easier it will be for us to keep track of her. What else?"

As Damien continued to fill him in on his impressions of Moerae, the shingled brown hair on the back of Paul's neck prickled. The shrink his ex-wife had insisted they go to see had labeled it a deep streak of paranoia combined with borderline schizophrenia. Inherited from his mother, the bastard had hypothesized. Psycho-babble bullshit to justify exorbitant fees, Paul had told him. He couldn't give a rat's ass what they called it, as long as it kept him from getting blindsided.

Paul suddenly realized he'd missed something Damien just said, and his radar system registered a noticeable blip. "Go back over what you just said. It sounded important."

"I said, at least she was perceptive enough to see what a tight meeting I ran," Damien answered.

The lady was good, smart enough to know that Damien and Joshua were alike. Paul had known for years that both were so hungry for praise, they left themselves wide open. Confident that Damien would mistake the gesture, Paul patted him on the knee. "She's got that right. Too bad some of the doctors aren't as smart."

Damien nodded and returned Paul's pat.

Paul stole a glance at the clock on Damien's immaculate desk. The straighter they stand, the easier they are to get around. In the hands of an expert such as himself, such predictability made manipulation a piece of cake. "So what's your bottom line? I've got to get to the O.R. Is she really dangerous?"

As always, when he solicited Damien's opinion, Damien sat up a bit straighter and paused before answering, "Like I said, she's a force to be reckoned with. But really dangerous? I don't think so. Actually, her theory about dysfunctional relationships among board members may serve us well."

Paul had already come to that conclusion but said, "Really! How so? Why do you say that?"

"Elementary, my dear Watson. It means you'll be able to keep a close watch on her and she may actually distract the board so they're less likely to catch wind of our extra-curricular little business venture."

Small fish swam in small ponds. He lusted for bigger things than milking some second-rate insurance company buying inside data. Their big-tittied lady friend might be very helpful in distracting Joshua. Then Paul could grab the whole nine yards.

He got up and stretched, glancing out Damien's window to the courtyard below. "Listen, I gotta run. But I think you're right on. I'll nose around with the other board guys. It looks like our lady has just met Rich Rosen," he said nodding toward the window.

From his own window, Peter Albert watched as Moerae walked across the courtyard on her way to him. He made a mental note to ask her about her bumping into Rich Rosen—particularly since, unless his eyes had deceived him, Damien had observed the same interaction. Hopefully they'd hit it off, for he sorely needed an ally he could trust.

Moments ago, a tall, soft-spoken young man with shoulder-length hair had just left his office. That meeting arose directly out of a strange sequence of events this past weekend that still had Peter amazed: It all began with his fourteen-year-old daughter's fit of rage over accidentally erasing her entire term paper. She knocked the mouse onto the floor and broke it into several pieces, requiring him to make a hurried trip to the computer store. Then by coincidence—no, he decided, *Providence*—he ran into Hal Mays, the friendly, talkative techno-geek who graciously agreed to come home with him and try to retrieve his daughter's paper.

A bit odd, Hal reminded Peter of the kind and gentle hippies from his bygone college days. But he knew his stuff, and he loved to talk about computers. As he explained retrieving lost data and "erased" files that weren't really erased, he wandered onto the subject of "trolls," sophisticated computer programs serving as watchdogs that silently record times, dates, and access codes of people who logged on to high-security computer systems.

The average computer user had no idea these programs even existed. Like the video cameras in banks or the new automatic cameras police now use to record traffic violations, these watch dogs can also record anyone's attempts to tamper with particular computer program logs. Peter's ears perked up when Hal explained that the only way into a troll's logs was by special access codes known only to the people who knew the watch dog existed.

143

When Peter asked Hal if he'd be interested in doing some investigative work on the computer system at his office, Hal had accepted enthusiastically. Peter said he just wanted to make sure C.C.A. had the most efficient back-up system for their computers.

At this point it would still require a good deal more digging before Hal could produce any of the details, but he was certain that C.C.A.'s massive hard drive showed signs that files had recently been erased. Hal was confident that he'd be able to retrieve a good bit of the lost content. With any luck, he'd also be able to identify which terminals had initiated the activity. Of course, thought Peter, one of those terminals will be Damien's.

To top it all off, Peter learned that Hal wouldn't even need to work at Peter's terminal to complete the job. He could do it from his own home. Peter was shocked. Any outsider with a few master keys could have access to all the corporation's closet skeletons.

Clicking heels on the linoleum outside his office pulled Peter's gaze from the window. He opened the door and Moerae towered over him. But when she thrust out her hand to him and grinned, Peter felt oddly as though they had known each other for years.

"Good morning, Moerae. It's a pleasure to meet you finally," Peter said.

"Peter, I've been looking forward to this meeting from the moment Joshua took me on. You must be someone special for him to have appointed you head of the finance review committee."

"Come in, come in! Don't stand on ceremony." He ushered her into his office. "Please excuse the chaos—but I assure you, it's *controlled* chaos," he continued, waving his hand into the air. "It must feel like night and day compared to the austerity you just came from."

She laughed. "You can say that again. Compared to your memorabilia, Damien's walls look like a prison cell." She pointed at the many framed diplomas and the prominently displayed family photographs hanging on the walls.

Peter laughed from his belly. "I'm getting an odd message here," he said, not letting go of her hand. "I have the distinct impression we're going to be very good friends, so let's get one thing out in the open right away: My wife tells me I remind people of their own son. I'm everyone's universal little boy. Maybe it's my size," he said rolling his eyes, "that brings out the mother in women."

Moerae threw her head back and laughed, and both of her hands virtually swallowed his. "If I'm as easy a read as that, I'm in danger of being embarrassed."

Peter squeezed her hand and released it, beaming. "Let's hope I'm the only one. Not all mind readers are friendly."

Further demonstrating how at-home Peter made her feel, Moerae poured herself a cup of coffee from the credenza without asking. "Hmmmm. Do I hear a warning bell?" Moerae turned to look at him quizzically.

Peter's shoulders relaxed a couple of inches away from his ears. The quickness of her mind, her ability to read subtle signals, ensured that she could play the verbal chameleon. If anyone thought they'd pulled the wool over her eyes, it would be because that was the impression she wanted them to have.

"I'm not sure," Peter said. "It's like exploratory surgery. You don't invade the body without having a pretty strong suspicion that something radical like cancer is attacking it. You just met with a likely candidate for being a carrier. What was your impression of our chief operating officer?"

Moerae snapped her fingers. "I meant to ask you before. How did you know I'd been to see Damien already? Are there any offices around here that aren't bugged?"

145

Peter nodded toward the big window overlooking the courtyards. "I happened to see you walking out of the administration building. The offices aren't literally bugged, but the grapevine is buzzing these days. I also saw you having a conversation with Rich Rosen, an interaction Damien was watching through his window, too, I might add. You weren't scheduled to talk with Rich, were you?"

She shook her mane of golden hair. "But I had a few extra minutes before our meeting and I couldn't resist playing my TLC game." She tilted her head and flashed Peter her best jack-o'-lantern smile.

"Okay. I'll bite. What's your 'tender love and care' game?"

"Very simple, really. I randomly stop a busy-looking physician and play 'the lost consultant'—TLC—needing directions. I can learn heaps about an organization's culture just by how helpful the response is."

Hesitantly, Peter asked, "And how did we do?"

"Quite well actually. After giving directions, he even offered to walk me over here, but I told him that wouldn't be necessary."

"I'm thrilled at our grade but I fear your results may be biased." Peter laughed. "For two reasons."

"Okay. Now it's my turn to bite," Moerae smiled back.

Peter held up two fingers. "One, your description has preceded you and, two, Rich is a healthy male."

Moerae shrugged, smiled, and shook her head in mock rue. "Guilty of gender-biased research, as charged."

"Enough," Peter said. "So how *did* you get on with Damien? I'm dying to find out."

"Well, I sure wouldn't leave him in the henhouse alone. But I must say, the cocks who rule the roost have drawn their share of his blood, and he doesn't suffer it lightly. He's a man to be reckoned with." Moerae moved toward the window overlooking the courtyard. She held up her coffee cup with both hands and sipped from it thoughtfully.

Peter came to stand next to her. Both of them stared out of the window as if hoping a divine sign would appear. "That's the understatement of the year. The man's potentially lethal and …

"Who is that man?" Moerae pointed excitedly toward the white-coated figure striding cockily across the courtyard below.

Peter tried to focus.

"That one," she said. "The one crushing the cigarette under his foot."

"You mean the tall, lanky one blowing smoke?" he asked. "Our chief anesthesiologist. His name is Paul Blake, but we call him Ichabod. Partly because of his build, but also because he's not exactly the sociable type. Like the way he persists in unhealthy habits—defying all medical knowledge. He's one of the few doctors who still smokes, and he delights in doing so openly. He's long since past caring what anyone thinks of him. Why do you ask?"

Moerae craned her erect neck. "He was headed into Damien's den of austerity just as I was leaving. I got the impression he was making a social call. It must've been a quick meeting, however."

Peter moved toward his desk. "That's Paul Blake, a slam-bam-thank-you-ma'am type of guy. But I'm not surprised." Reaching into his pocket, Peter removed a small key ring. Sitting down at his desk, he unlocked the bottom right-hand drawer and lifted out a metal box. It contained a full dossier of information on Paul Blake, which he'd painstakingly culled himself.

"From everything I've discovered in the last few weeks, Dr. Blake is one of the primary hot spots in the war we've got brewing."

"Do you have one of these on me, too?" Moerae asked, play-fully tapping the dossier.

He winked at her. "Your reputation also precedes you. Besides," he said, turning serious, "I wouldn't have taken on this assignment if I didn't have complete faith in Joshua's judgment and motivations."

"I didn't mean to suggest otherwise, Peter. But if you're feeling the need to defend Joshua, you must have reason to be concerned."

Peter cleared his throat. "He's under a tremendous amount of stress and I needn't tell you how much this place means to him. That's not a healthy combination when it comes to promoting objectivity and clear-headedness."

A computer disk sat at the bottom of the folder and she pointed to it. "Is it safe to keep your hard copy and the computer disk in the same place?" Moerae asked.

"You're good! That little computer disk may hold some missing pieces vital to this puzzle we're trying to put together. Right now, let me just say it's a long shot I'm following."

"This from the man who said, 'You don't invade the body without a pretty strong suspicion.' I'll let you go with that. You can fill me in when you're ready." Moerae winked in an exaggerated fashion. "I'll need some help scripting the key parts of my tête-à-tête with the board. What's the easiest way for me to arrange a dress rehearsal?"

"Let me think for a minute." Peter paced in front of the window.

He watched the clouds moving across the blue sky, their whiteness like the cream in the center of luscious cupcakes. He replayed part of an earlier conversation he'd had with Joshua, in which they'd agreed not to involve Joshua with preliminary feedback. But he had referred specifically to the financial part of his review.

Could he justify excluding Joshua from the planning sessions with Moerae? Could he risk another kind of 'star chamber'? He continued to pace until he turned back to face Moerae.

"Why don't you give me a call next week when you feel ready for a dry run? We can get together for a drink and play it out a bit. I may bring along another colleague," he said, thinking of Ross. "Just to keep you and me honest. How's that sound to you?"

She nodded. "We'll need a couple of hours. How much advance notice do you need to set up such a meeting?"

Peter shrugged. "Just give me a day. For what I have in mind, it won't be difficult to set it up. Joshua's busy these days and unless you feel strongly otherwise, I'd be inclined not to bother him with the boredom of a rehearsal."

"No, I think that's a great idea. Heck, he's paying for it. We should save the opening-night show for him."

They smiled at one another, a hint of conspiracy flashing in her amber eyes.

Moerae stood. "I'm ready to go. My lunch appointment is with Mary Howard. She seems a dear, and good as gold as far as information is concerned. Is there anyone else in particular you think I should touch base with as I sniff around?"

"I don't remember seeing Kathy Marshall on your list. If she isn't, try to make some time to see her. She's in touch with much of what goes on around the place and she'll help balance the boys' club stories you'll be hearing."

"Thanks, Peter. With Kathy's and den mother Howard's insights, I feel more assured that I'll get a balanced *agender*." She giggled at the face Peter made at her pun.

Yes, indeed. They were going to be real allies.

Eleven

Moerae looked out the window from her apartment on Lakeshore Drive. A rare early summer day in Chicago. The smog was so thin she could almost see the Country Club where the C.C.A. board retreat would begin this evening.

Maybe the good weather was an omen. With lots of help from Ross Benson, Peter Albert, and Jane, she'd worked harder to prepare for this retreat than for any other. Only two items left to do, which she had scribbled on the yellow refrigerator note. Call a limo and call Ruth. The last piece of the puzzle would be an up-to-date reading of Joshua's frame of mind.

Over the past week, Moerae had uncovered a host of aches and pains throbbing in C.C.A. None of them in and of itself was particularly unusual or critical. In fact, most of the challenges facing C.C.A. told a familiar story.

Simply put, C.C.A. needed to grow up. The organization displayed all the characteristics of a spoiled child who believed the world owed it something. The doctors especially would have to stop playing their fraternity games, which included squabbling over money, time off, and trips to professional meetings in exotic locations, that served no other purpose but to squander enormous amounts of time and energy. Whoever had the longest reach and the quickest hands grabbed the goodies first.

Humility wasn't a highly valued asset anywhere else in the business world either. Most successful professionals in all walks of life shared the same tendency to take their achievements personally.

The fundamental principle that guided all of Moerae's thinking was that businesses were made up *of* human beings, *by* human beings, and *for* them. Therefore, it followed that businesses exhibited all of the human strengths and weaknesses, patterns of decay and growth, and potential for creativity or failure of the people who made them up.

Unfortunately, most businesses seemed to be stuck at the mental level of precocious adolescents. Their public relations departments cloak this immaturity with terms such as *human resources* or *personnel*. They invent a whole new jargon to distance management from the real people who worked for them. CEOs talk about *downsizing* or *re-engineering* as if that were as simple as shrinking a sweater that had gotten pulled out of shape.

To Moerae, downsizing was like performing massive surgery without anesthesia. Moerae prayed that today she'd be able to show the board at C.C.A. the importance of treating human beings as sacred gifts, not simply as another kind of commodity—an asset to be managed.

It was time to get on the stick. Moerae pushed one of her phone's automatic dialing buttons for the limo service. A mechanical voice asked her to hold. Moerae sighed. Every time she called A-One she was put on hold before she could open her mouth.

"Excuse me for keeping you waiting," the voice came back, surprising her with its pleasantness. "How may I help you?"

"I need a limo at Lakeside Towers North at about five p.m. I'm going to the Outer Loop Country Club."

"That's on the other side of the city, ma'am. Our drivers have alerted us that there are some very bad accidents on the Beltway this afternoon. May I ask when you need to be there?"

Moerae grinned into the receiver and let her shoulders fall from their tensed-up position around her ears. That'll teach you to assume the worst, she thought. It was always so nice to hear a real person on the other end of the line—and one with helpful advice. A four forty-five pick up would still give her time to call Ruth.

"That'll be fine. And thanks again for the suggestion."

"My pleasure, ma'am. Have a nice party."

As soon as she disconnected, her call-waiting button flashed.

"Hello, Dr. King's office," she said.

"My, that sounds so official," Ruth's warm voice teased.

"Well, I'm getting ready to go into the lion's den, so I'm sharpening all my swords. I was just going to call you and get a last-minute update on how Joshua is doing. I've only got about fifteen minutes before my limo will be here, though."

"Great minds work alike," Ruth said. "Joshua is … well, Joshua. As far as I can tell, the retreat is stirring up nothing unusual. For him, at least."

Moerae stopped arranging the papers in her C.C.A. folder. Ruth's voice sounded suspiciously neutral. "For him, at least?" What is it you're not saying? Is someone *else* feeling stirred up?"

Moerae could hear Ruth rustling in her desk chair. "I'm not sure. I know how focused you'll need to be to manage the retreat. You don't need any unnecessary distractions coming from me. Especially since they're so … so vague."

Moerae allowed a little sternness into her voice. "Ruth, let me be the judge of what I can handle and how. You're worrying me. It's not like you to be vague. A smart psychologist like you. It must be something close to your heart, to make you blind like that. If you really want to know what I don't need to be

---

153

worrying about, it's whether there are any land mines planted in my path that I'm unaware of. If you have misgivings of any kind, I want you to say them to me. Out with it, woman."

"Well, you know Peter's been heading up the special finance review committee."

"Yeah, he told me he was following a few hunches and would fill me in as things developed."

"And Mary happened to tell me just the other day," Ruth continued, "that she was in the office on Sunday catching up on some paperwork. Peter and some computer expert he's hired were also holed up in Peter's office the entire time she was in."

"Ruth honey, there's nothing strange about that. That place is lousy with workaholics. Now listen, I love you dearly, but could you please get to the point?"

"Mary said that Peter could see that she was at her desk, but he never once, during the entire day, came out to even say hello. That's not like Peter, Moerae."

Moerae's antenna vibrated again, this time strongly. This wasn't a phone call about Mary feeling put out by Peter's not saying hello. This was about something frightening her good friend, Ruth. Her intuition guided her: Go gently here. Don't let her bolt.

"Hmm, you're right," she responded, "I don't think that's like Peter either, not from what I know of him. He must've been really wrapped up in something to have shunned Mary for the entire day. Any idea what it was?"

All in one breath Ruth blurted, "I don't know what it is either, but I agree completely. He's onto something and it isn't sitting too well, I can tell."

As lightly as she could Moerae said, "Okay, Detective Caliban. Tell me what your keen intuitive nose has smelled."

"Well, you know how close Peter and Joshua are."

"Like father and son."

"Exactly, Moerae. That's what made a phone call from Peter so strange this morning. Peter called me, claiming just to say hello. But he spent half the conversation asking me all kinds of questions about how Joshua's feeling these days."

"And what did Peter say when you asked him about it?"

"He immediately back-pedaled. I mean, what he said made perfect sense, but there was something … something almost ominous. It was the *way* he said it that made me nervous," Ruth finished.

Moerae nestled the phone under her ear and rubbed the sweat from the palm of her hand. "Ominous. That's a pretty strong word. But you're still not quite giving it to me. You know, my mind-reading ability has gotten really rusty. Do you think you could just say it, Ruth? Help me out here."

The laugh over the phone came as a welcome relief. "You're right, Moerae, I'm probably making a mountain out of a molehill. I guess I'm a bit anxious myself about how things will go at the retreat. It's an important meeting."

Moerae laughed back. "Tell me about it! But quick, tell me what Peter said! The lobby is buzzing me. My limo must be here."

"Oh, Peter was wanting to know how Joshua's stress level was these days. Those were his words exactly. And then, get this. He says, 'You know how proud Joshua is. He tries to do everything by himself. I just want to be sure we're doing everything we can to help him.' He really is hard to help, isn't he, Moerae?"

"He'll be doubly hard to help if I don't get there on time." Moerae laughed again to relax Ruth. Her antenna told her that Ruth was truly on to something. But now she had to disentangle herself from this conversation to dash downstairs. "I make my presentation right after dinner. Don't worry. All my instincts tell me the operation will be a success. I'll call you from the club if I can get a minute to breathe. Or tonight when I get home, if it isn't too late or I'm not a basket case."

"Good luck, Moerae." Ruth was quiet for a moment. Moerae could almost see her friend fingering the tiny fertility goddess figure that always sat on her office desk. "I love you."

Moerae would bet money that she'd interpreted Ruth's hesitation correctly. Ruth had just passed the weight of responsibility for her loved one squarely onto Moerae's shoulders. "I love you, too," she said, and hung up.

On the ride over, she rehashed the conversation. No doubt about it. Ruth's intuition had hooked on something very real. Where there was smoke, there was bound to be fire. Peter was a hungry lion on the hunt. Moerae suspected that his anxiety probably encompassed more than just the flames he saw raging all around Joshua. His concern also seemed to include Joshua himself. What complexities lay hidden in Joshua's shadow?

The limo pulled up under the massive stone arch at the entryway to the prestigious Outer Loop Country Club. Given the circumstances, the antebellum ambiance of the club might have intimidated Moerae or at least distracted her. But the building was familiar. She'd been there many times before.

The uniformed doorman reached down to the door of the limo and greeted her with a warm smile. "Welcome back, Dr. King."

"Thank you," Moerae replied, touched that he remembered her. "Can you tell me where the C.C.A. board meeting is being held?"

"Certainly. It's in the Trophy Room just down the main hall. As far as I know, they've all arrived."

She'd planned to be one of the last to arrive so that the tone of the gathering would have already built up when she walked in. She had only a few seconds to sniff the air from the doorway, but that was all she would need. Mary Howard caught her eye and telegraphed a smile so discreetly that Roger Rosen, with whom she was in conversation, never even turned to see whose entry had distracted her. Ross and Peter, their heads together over a small table, were talking animatedly.

Damien and Paul leaned against the bar, washing down handfuls of potato chips with great gulps of beer. Moerae watched them intently before Damien noticed her presence. A small shudder ran through her. In spite of her distance from them, the disdain and mistrust burning hot in his eyes could have singed her skin. Those two were strange bedfellows.

Damien's lips mouthed her arrival to Paul who immediately turned his back to her. Ichabod Crane. Great name. An interesting composition of opposites made up Paul Blake. His anger could blaze like a furnace, but his outward demeanor could chill you to the bone. He'd given her the coldest reception of all and presented a formidable force. Oh, how dearly she would love to stuff his head into the noose. But she planned simply to give him all the rope he needed to do the job himself. She smiled to Damien who was ostentatiously waving hello. The same goes for you, my friend, she thought.

Joshua, Scott, and Jane stepped into the room from the veranda. Joshua lit up when he saw her, warming her heart. She started down the steps to meet him.

Joshua came across the room to greet her alone. "Hello, Moerae. It's very good to see you," he said, reaching his hand out to her. "You know everyone here by now."

"Hello, Joshua. I just arrived. Sorry I'm a little late. The Beltway was terrible."

"You looked like a general surveying the battlefield standing up there at the door. You're obviously very skilled at making entrances," Joshua said. He looked into her eyes, which were level with his.

Joshua's happiness to see her seemed sincere. His arm on hers felt natural. Their ease with one another buoyed her optimism for what the evening could bring. He was enjoying this unique circumstance immensely. Somehow it made their confederacy seem ordained, as if by divine providence.

He steered her toward the bar. "What'll you have?"

"Soda water with lemon, although I'd prefer an Absolut martini," she said. "But I have to keep my wits about me, as I'm the only one who can't afford to fall asleep after dinner."

"I very much doubt that anyone will be falling asleep during your opening remarks. Everyone's read through your preliminary analysis and I'm sure there'll be a lot of questions. You aren't worried, are you?" he teased.

"Do I give that impression?" Moerae asked, slightly startled. "No, I'm not anxious about this evening. Just … alert. There are a few things I would've liked to ask Peter, but I'm sure they can wait."

Joshua's forehead curled and he tilted his chin down. She chastised herself. She must be more nervous than she was aware, to react so quickly to a teasing remark.

"Anything I can help with?" he asked.

She wished she could plumb Joshua's mind as easily as he seemed to navigate her thoughts. "No, no, rest assured. I have plenty of material for this evening's entertainment." She squeezed his hand and smiled.

"Well, then, you can start making your rounds with everyone. I'll bring you a soda, and grab a few hors d'oeuvres before the vultures scoff them all. Here's the man himself," Joshua said as Peter moved to join them. "And he looks like he needs a refill, too.

Joshua left and Moerae smiled and asked, "Any last minute words of wisdom before I get up there and open my mouth?"

"You'll do fine." Peter squeezed her arm reassuringly. "I'd go a little easy on the troops, however. Several people have been fighting a bad virus the past few days."

158

"Troops" and "virus" set off Moerae's inner alarm. Ruth's intuition had been right on. Peter's exploratory probing on Sunday must have uncovered something serious in the computer network. But Moerae wouldn't know how serious until after they'd finished tonight and she could speak with Peter in private. For the time being, she'd have to tread lightly. She could be neither so tentative as to confuse Joshua nor so inflammatory as to enrage Damien or Paul. Her best bet would be to avoid exacerbating the widening gulf between Joshua, Ross, and Peter on one side and Damien, Paul and Scott on the other.

She nodded and Joshua started to move the group into the adjoining dining room. Moerae sat between Joshua and Mary Howard. Moerae had barely tasted the crème brûleé before she was aware of Joshua's brief introduction of her and his hopes that her report would set the tone for the important strategic planning they'd begin tomorrow. She focused all her energies on centering herself, reaching inside to that expansive place of stillness that provided her spiritual strength. By the time Joshua had finished, Moerae was clear. She got up and went to the speaker's lectern feeling completely at ease.

"I assume that you have each carefully studied the report I prepared based on my preliminary diagnosis of C.C.A.'s state of human health," she began, adopting the formal tone Ross and Peter had agreed would be most effective. "I'd like to begin by asking you to bear with me for just a moment to consider the four following statements:

"True or false: All patients can be healed but not cured.

"True or false: Interpersonal staff infections can be as lethal as staph infections.

"True or false: Boardroom behavior impacts treatment room care.

"True or false: TLC, tender love and care, adds to both profitability and quality care."

Moerae paused and waited, standing straight and tall while she drew every person's attention to her. The silence and measured breathing around the table assured her that she had created the air of expectancy she'd hoped for. Not even Paul resisted looking up from his moody study of the dessert plate. She picked up her glass of water, not so much out of thirst, but more to have an excuse to steal a quick glance at Joshua. His arms folded on his belly said that he, too, was impressed with the command she'd managed to generate within just a few seconds' time.

Moerae laughed with real delight, dissolving instantly all the stiffness in the air. "It's been a long time since any of us were in school, but I'm sure everyone in this room got one hundred percent on this little exam. We all recognize and accept the essential truth of each of those statements. They're the truths that distinguish the difference between car dealerships and care dealerships."

Damien raised his hand. "You made a lot of that distinction in your report. If I remember correctly, you warned us that without healing, health care organizations become assembly lines, and," he looked down at a note, "interpersonal toxicity of any kind is infectious and detrimental to a healthy practice." Damien looked up again. "I must say, what confuses me is your linking those dynamics to boardroom behavior."

"I'm so glad you brought up this point right away," Moerae said brightly. As an adversary Damien was an antagonist into whom she could sink her teeth. "You're probably familiar with the Midland Airline debacle in the winter of '95. If you remember, the plane went down into the water off LaGuardia. The pilots were in an impossible bind. The appalling weather conditions forced a critical choice: On one hand, they could cancel all flights until conditions were less hazardous. The pilots knew that if they failed to follow F.A.A. safety standards, they'd bring severe disapproval down on their heads from management and possibly even dismissal. But on the other hand, they were obligated to fulfill their duty to delivering service to their customers.

"In hindsight, we've collected considerable evidence to indicate that it was the way *management* dealt with the conflict between quality and quantity that directly contributed to the accident. In other words, their general philosophy tended to side with choosing numbers over safety in their business decisions."

Scott looked like a school kid needing to hit the head. "But the Midland board members don't fly the planes! That's like blaming the Cubs manager every time one of those turkeys on the field blows a play."

Moerae winced. Could the guy be any more inane? "What would you say was your responsibility as a board member, Dr. MacDonald?" she asked politely.

"More to the point," Paul Blake said, strumming his fingers loudly on the table, "You said yourself that we're a *care* dealership. How does what we do around the boardroom table ever affect the factory floor?"

"Thank you, Paul, for redirecting me. I should've couched my example in medical terms. If I could impose on your patience for a moment longer, I'll explain." She watched Paul closely. He was an oily one, an emotional chameleon. She had expected his natural rancor to surface at some point in the evening and was satisfied it had done so early.

"One of the probes I often use to diagnose the health of a care dealership goes like this: Imagine that your loved one has a severe or life-threatening illness. You know that C.C.A. has the technical personnel and equipment to handle the case. Let's assume, further, that all the physicians available have the proper board certification and could be considered to have equal levels of skill.

"Now ask yourself: How comfortable would you feel if the physician managing the case were to be assigned on a purely random basis? And then ask, are there any specific physicians in C.C.A. whom you would *not* choose? Who would you want to protect your loved one from?"

Mary sighed and dropped her head to her chin. Roger leaned back on the legs of his chair. Joshua and Peter shot quick glances at Paul and Scott.

Ross straightened his unwrinkled tie and leaned forward. "It sounds like what you're driving at, Moerae, is that the chemistry between patient and provider is very important to the quality of care given. But I must say that I still don't see the connection to the boardroom."

Moerae answered without batting an eye. "In my experience, I've found that in organizations where there is significant distrust of what you have very astutely labeled 'chemistry,' there are senior executives who have great difficulty being honest and direct with one another."

The room was growing tense. In an attempt to ease the mounting pressure, Jane spoke up: "Let me try to help clarify here, because I think this point is fundamental to what Dr. King is asking us to consider." Moerae nodded and Jane continued, "Just last week, two landmark cases were tried that have profound and frightening implications for industry at large and health care in particular. The Supreme Court of Colorado ruled that an employer could be held accountable for the quality of the human process by which a performance appraisal was conducted. In plain words, it isn't simply the bad news, but the manner in which bad news is delivered that's at issue. Is it humane or cruel in its effects?"

"Jesus," Peter said, "with the climate in this country today being so litigation-prone, we could get sued simply because of the way we tell a patient the results of their diagnosis!"

Damien stiffened his back. Joshua winced and shook his head.

"It gets worse, and even more to Moerae's point," Jane continued. "The Supreme Court of Texas recently upheld a lower court ruling that allowed a hospital patient to sue an entire department for complicity in malpractice. It was found that many of the staff had shared their concerns about the specific doctor in question ... with everyone but that doctor. They had knowledge of what was going on, and their silence about it made them complicit in the doctor's wrongful practices."

"I've been trying to tell them for years," Damien said, his beady eyes about to pop out of his head from his earnestness. "I told them they'd better get rid of the bad apples before they spoil the whole barrel!"

"The first barrel we have to clean up sits on our boardroom table," Joshua said. "That's the very table from which we presumably operate as an organization. I gather that you asked those chemistry questions of people in C.C.A.," he said to Moerae.

Moerae nodded, hoping Joshua remembered her commitment not to associate any comments she made with specific individual's names.

Roger Rosen cleared his throat. "I have some very serious concerns about the implications of what you've proposed. If we were to follow your recommendations, it would ultimately turn the organization upside down. It's one thing to ask patients how satisfied they are with aspects of the regular services we provide such as scheduling, waiting time, et cetera, but what you're proposing is that we allow patients to define the *quality* of the care they receive."

"I apologize if I gave that impression, Dr. Rosen. Only a peer among a doctor's colleagues, one who is an equally skilled and highly trained professional, could judge the technical quality of the care a patient receives. Even that assumes that these

---

163

professionals are willing to give each other clear, direct, honest feedback."

Damien pointed a menacing finger in the air. "At the risk of sounding like a broken record, how long have we been talking about the need for a performance appraisal system that includes the doctors?"

"To clarify the point that Dr. Rosen raised, my proposal doesn't refer to the quality of the technical care a patient receives. It concerns specifically the *human* quality of care given by every person with whom a patient comes in contact. Do they get respect? Dignity? Empathy? With respect to these dimensions of quality, the patient is, and will remain, the final authority."

"It makes logical sense to me, Moerae, but I can imagine the logistical problems such a philosophy would create," Peter said. "You're talking about allowing, in fact encouraging, patients to give their providers direct, honest feedback on how they need to be treated. Keeping track of these needs would be a nightmare."

Moerae nodded. This was one of the leading questions planted at strategically important points in her presentation that she, Peter, and Ross had planned. "The major obstacle is not logistical in nature. You have no difficulty keeping track of every aspirin a patient gets or billing him for it. Call Dominos and, if you've ordered a pizza in the past year, they can tell you what the toppings were." Moerae paused for effect. "The point, gentlemen, is that the way patients get treated mirrors the way employees treat one another. I believe the major obstacle is our ego. It's human nature to resist being held accountable for the consequences of our actions, for the effect we have on others."

A flush appeared along Paul's raised cheekbones. "I don't agree with Peter. I don't even think it makes logical sense. It's insane to imagine that everyone in the organization is a caregiver. You want my behavior to be judged by the nurse to whom

I give orders? Hell, if she ever criticized me, I'd boot her out so fast she wouldn't know what hit her."

"Judging from the turnover among nurse anesthetists, it doesn't appear as if most of them wait around long enough for your boot to make contact," Joshua stated acidly. "I can't say it's been comfortable, Moerae," he continued, "but I believe your comments and your report will give us a running start tomorrow in our planning session. I'll call you the first part of next week and let you know what our decision is concerning your specific next step proposals. Does anyone have any further questions for Dr. King?"

"I say we carry on the discussion around the bar," Peter offered. "We've got a full day's work tomorrow."

Twelve

Joshua walked purposefully down the corridor toward his office. Crises always seemed to come at once. Like a tightly knit school of sardines, distinguishing one from another was sometimes impossible. To try to solve one often meant getting bogged down in them all. And the ones given by someone else were the most slippery, hard to grasp, and harder still to hold on to.

His colleagues were growing restless again. As the staff bitched and moaned, it seemed that patients had more complaints, too. The more recalcitrant the docs became, the more he wanted to scream at them. They wasted so much time complaining. If they would only convert that energy to taking care of business, they wouldn't be facing pay cuts.

An airplane taking off from O'Hare roared overhead. Its noise penetrated the building and Joshua's consciousness, diverting his attention to the story Moerae had told him about TransCentral Airlines. It was the same airline that had taken the lives of Ruth's parents, the same airline about which a government investigation had concluded: "The safety of the passengers in an airplane was being adversely effected by the wall of mistrust and suspicion that had been built between management and the union."

Joshua tried to shake it off, but the point kept spinning around and around in his brain.

The lunch hour was usually a time Joshua looked forward to so he could catch his breath from the intensity of the morning. But as he got closer to his office, the back of his throat tasted sour, and his skin prickled unpleasantly. He was on his way to meet Peter and get his first report on the meetings of the finance review committee. Peter had begged off assisting him on the last two procedures this morning, which he did only in the case of a real emergency.

"We just need a few hours to pin down some last-minute details so I can have the headlines ready for you over lunch today. Nothing for you to worry about."

"You're a very poor liar, Peter," Joshua had said.

Peter had cleared his throat and said nothing in reply.

As he came up to Mary's desk, she was taking a phone message but didn't even give him a cursory glance over the top of her bifocals.

"I could swear I smell something burning," he said. "And I have a nasty feeling it's not from the electrical storms threatening the rest of Chicago. Has the phone been burning up the wires this morning? Never mind," he said, as Mary stonewalled him. "You're not going to talk, I can see that. You look exactly like a Vegas card dealer." Joshua watched her trying to sort the thick stack of pink phone slips.

"Trying to deal you a winning hand from this mess won't be easy, unless you feel like you can draw to an inside straight," Mary said.

He laughed. "Remind me never to play poker with you, woman. What have you got?"

Mary started her catalog of messages with the name of the president of the Bar Association.

"Virgil Carter called. He was pretty closed-mouthed, wouldn't give me any details, but he wanted to know if you had any comment on the interesting new malpractice twist C.C.A. was facing."

The hairs on the back of his neck bristled. "Tell me more."

"No sooner do I hang up on him, than the producer of the six o'clock CBS news program calls with essentially the same question. I called Jane Sherwood immediately. Her secretary said she was out of the office but that she'd page her. Jane phoned me just a few seconds before you came in. She said she couldn't talk but that you should just follow the normal procedure. She'll be back by five-thirty and needs to see you before you go home."

"I get the message." When Jane advised him to follow normal procedure, she meant he should talk to no one without her being present. And Jane rarely needed to see him before he went home.

"So, the calls from Virgil and CBS are all on hold. What other goodies have you got?"

"Let's see, Dr. King called. If you have a minute over lunch she'd like an update on how the retreat turned out. And Little Boy Blue was on the horn to you. He said he had some good news for you. The rest of the stuff I can take care of for now."

Joshua quietly stroked his beard. So Ashton Simons was trying to reach him. When Big Blue called and said it was good news, Joshua translated it as problematic. If the news did turn out to be good for C.C.A., it was only because it was better for Big Blue.

Given the kind of morning it had been and what the afternoon appeared to have in store, Joshua decided to call Moerae first. He needed something to offset the acid bubbling through his gut. Shit. No "babies" left in the drawer. He could've sworn he'd stopped by pharmacy just yesterday. Hell, he thought he could even recall a conversation with an inquisitive tech who hadn't recognized him.

Hearing the solid timbre of Moerae's voice lifted his spirits immediately. He gave her a brief update. While the group had

---

seemed open to discussing her follow-up proposals, they were of no mind to take any immediate action. He hadn't expected support from Paul or Scott, but even Peter, Roger, and Ross seemed to be marking time. Maybe they were right. Decisions were better left until the financial review was finished. He'd find out soon enough what the gist of it was.

"Listen, Moerae, Peter has just arrived," Joshua said into his phone as he saw Peter open his door and bustle into his office, carrying an attaché case and clipboard. Turned down lips accentuated the dour look on his otherwise cherub baby face. "From the look on his face, I'd say he's not a happy camper. I'll keep in touch as things develop. It's only a matter of time before we'll need you." He hung up the phone. "That good?" Joshua said in mock jest as he pushed his chair out from behind his desk and stood up. Joshua never took bad news sitting down.

Peter, on the other hand, delivered bad news seated. People wouldn't hit a little guy that was down, he explained when Joshua teased him about the habit. He settled himself onto the couch as Joshua began to pace slowly. "It's mixed," Peter said.

With customary brevity, Peter summarized his findings.

Hal Mays' research into the computer system had cast some very dark shadows over Damien. In fact, they were so serious that Peter had decided to alert Joshua even before he met with Ross and Roger.

Peter passed a piece of paper to Joshua. The graphs revealed a disturbing story. Two of the three figures were sloping gently but unmistakably upward. These confirmed that billable income was well above overhead expenses. C.C.A.'s business was booming. But the third figure was faintly ominous. It plotted the payments made by Big Blue. In any twelve-month period, it made a straight line. Over longer periods, it looked like a series of very shallow steps always striving to catch up with the other two curves—revenues and expenses—but never quite drawing even.

Peter's explanation for why this was happening was simple. In busy times like the one they were currently enjoying, the harder they ran, the faster and farther behind they fell. This was because the greater the volume of business C.C.A. did, the bigger a line of credit they needed to draw from the bank. The more money the bank advanced them, the more interest C.C.A. was charged. And the more interest they owed, the harder it was to borrow money.

Joshua took one more disdainful look at the graphs and dropped it into Peter's lap. "It's a goddamn financial treadmill. Why in the hell hasn't anyone on the board caught on to it before now?"

Peter shrugged. "You know docs, Joshua. Most of them won't even periodically balance their own checking accounts."

Peter dropped the sheet into his attaché case and snapped it shut. Joshua thought he'd seen another folder marked Personal Mays Stuff. Strange of Peter not to have pulled it out, but he decided not to ask about it.

Joshua poured himself a cup of coffee. "Ashton Simons, the pig behind this gig, called this morning. Mary said he had some good news."

"I don't need to tell you, Joshua, that most money traders play the same game. Your banker tells you that your deposit can't be drawn against for a few days, then he deposits the funds in a government short-term money market for the interim. It might earn only pennies on the dollar, but when hundreds of millions of dollars are involved, it turns into substantial manna from heaven. We've been really pumping up the receivables," he continued. "The float gap must be getting so wide that Ashton is afraid that we'd catch it ourselves."

Joshua nodded. "I'll be able to extract more than enough from our keeper of the blood bank to settle the score. What really bothers me is that Damien's been involved in what's clearly a conflict of interest for such a long time. I can't believe he doesn't know about it. He's a member of their board, if you remember. I really trusted the guy to be more careful about this."

"I only got wind of this one yesterday, so I'd like to let go of it for the moment. I've got some more digging to do. I'm afraid this could be just the tip of the iceberg. Give me until tomorrow, and I'll have more details."

"Why does talking about icebergs make me think of the Titanic?" Joshua was only half joking. His anxiety level raised several notches when Peter squirmed in his chair.

"Well, I happened to call Mr. Wong the other day, partly to see how he was doing. By the way, he said that he hadn't forgotten you. He'll be sending the letter Mrs. Wong had promised you directly."

Joshua's felt the pounding in his temple signaling a rise in his blood pressure. But he knew that his patience with Peter would always be rewarded with a valuable insight. That was Peter's way.

"I also called to thank him for his prompt payment of his wife's bill. When I was looking over our recent receivables, I noticed that he'd paid the entire thing. Now I know they're not poor, but this surprised me. He also said to thank you for the discount he assumed you must have given him. If Mrs. Wong were still here, she wouldn't hear of it, he said. So he went ahead and paid the full amount. That's seventy-five thousand dollars! In a matter of days!"

"I did ask Damien to see what he could do for them. I'm glad to hear that he did." Joshua fidgeted. When was Peter going to get to the point?

"So I asked him, kind of casually, if he wouldn't have preferred some kind of payment schedule to lighten the load. He said no, and explained why. It seems that when Mrs. Wong almost died on the table a few years ago, a company called Care, Inc. contacted the family."

Suddenly Joshua's stomach lurched. He stopped pacing to listen intently. For several minutes Peter described what Care, Inc. provided their customers. With each passing minute, Joshua's sense of nausea increased.

"The Wongs had planned to leave the hundred thousand to the kids," Peter continued, "but when it became apparent that she might need another operation, the family held a meeting. Mr. Wong said it was, and I quote 'kind of like one of your board meetings, Doc.' They decided unanimously that one more day with Mama was worth all the money in the world."

"That's about as far from one of our board decisions as you can get!" Joshua snorted. "Listen, I'm trying to be patient. You know how badly I felt about losing Mrs. Wong, but where are you leading me with this story?"

"It's only a hypothesis at this point," Peter said, "but I'm pretty sure Damien's been selling patient information."

Joshua clenched his teeth. Peter's attempt to soften the blow hadn't worked. "He's been what!"

"I know this is infuriating to both of us, Joshua, but hear me out will you."

Joshua pressed his lips together and nodded.

"With my computer expert's help, I've learned that C.C.A.'s computers are linked together in such a way that its network functions much like a human brain. Just as different parts of the brain can communicate with other parts, these computer terminals can communicate with each other. Anyone with the correct code, and Damien in particular, could access patient records from any terminal in the facility and send information from that terminal to any other."

Joshua rubbed his fists together. "That makes me sick. It was Damien himself who sold us on this ingenious system. I've been stabbed in the back twice, first by my own board members and then by that ingrate. Why, I've even defended him against all comers!"

Peter rose and ran his pudgy fingers through his uncombed towhead. "Pisses me off, too. Damien has abused the privileges of the system by requesting that a specific group of patient records be networked to the terminal at his desk!"

Joshua shook his head. Hard. "Yeah, but Peter, doesn't Damien need those kinds of records to deal with patient complaints?"

Peter held out his hands palms up and shrugged. "That was my first reaction too, Joshua. Hal Mays did a few quick studies for me. Some of the records Damien requested were returned to the central file in a matter of hours. Others were kept for several days. Here's the clincher. The longer a patient's file sat in Damien's computer, the more likely the patient's condition was to become terminal.

"What made me suspicious was ... " Peter stopped and cleared his throat.

Joshua raised his eyes at the pause. Something hard was coming.

"When I saw Mrs. Wong's name on the list, I got really suspicious and dug deeper. Damien first asked for her file the day after her operation two years ago, then again just the other day."

"How in the hell do you get that kind of information?" Joshua bellowed.

"Hal knows our system like the back of his hand. He helped design it years ago. The computer's watchdog systems work like trolls," Peter said. "Most of the time, they sleep quietly under the bridges that link the terminals in a network. They log traffic. On this day, at this time, so-and-so carried such-and-such across this bridge."

"Most of the time?" Joshua had stopped pacing and stood perfectly still, facing Peter with all of his senses alert.

"Not everyone has the code that gives access to the watchdog functions. Without the code, there's no way to read what the log entries are. If anyone tries to edit the logs, an alarm goes off and wakes up the troll. The troll is a jealous creature. Just like in the fairy tales, trolls don't like having someone walking over their bridges carrying off their logs. Without the code, it's better to let sleeping dogs lie."

Joshua turned his back to Peter, bit his lip and casually wiped a bead of sweat that had formed on his brow. He tried to ignore the possibility that somebody was watching his own editing of pharmacy logs. "Damien's the only dog who's been lying! Are you telling me that another watchdog might be watching the first one?"

"I don't know yet, Joshua. Hal has to do some more digging. But even if he doesn't find one, and he's confident he will, Damien still has some fancy explaining to do."

"And he's going to do it this afternoon," Joshua said, reaching for his intercom.

"Yes, Dr. Caliban," Mary answered immediately.

"Call Damien's office. Tell his secretary to make certain that he doesn't leave today until he hears from me personally. Is that clear?"

"Yes, sir!"

"Do things really come in threes or are you finished being the bearer of good cheer for the time being?" He steeled himself for the worst.

"This is the last one for now. And it really has me confused. When Hal alerted me to the trolls, I did some checking into what

---

175

other access codes Damien might have. I started with all the logical choices, and I honestly don't know what possessed me to snoop into the one I did. Maybe I was thinking about how my daughter, Sarah, never seems to be able to remember which of her allergy pills she's taken or when. Anyway, it occurred to me to check the pharmacy. And I discovered one of Damien's access codes is for the inventory control program in the pharmacy."

Joshua sat down behind his desk. He started to reach into his drawer but stopped, remembering his Valium supply was gone. He took a deep breath to try to calm the alarm bells going off in his head. "That's perfectly logical. It's his responsibility to double-check the actual inventory against the amount the supplier says they shipped."

"That was my first reaction too," Peter replied gently. He paused briefly, a discomfited look on his face. "But I happened to be down in pharmacy the other day to pick up some pills for Sarah. The pharmacist on duty apologized that they had accidentally dropped and broken the bottle. I told her I'd wait for them to refill it since I was on my way home anyway. The next thing I know, she's filling out this special form, a drug destruction form. It's part of Damien's system."

Joshua played with a pen, flicking the ballpoint on and off.

"According to the troll, Damien's entries into the log didn't match up with either the delivery dates from our suppliers or the specifics of the DDs," Peter went on. "What do you make of that?"

Joshua's mind raced, looking for a way to bend the finger of blame from casting its dark shadow in his direction. He banged his fist on top of his desk. "It sounds like a pretty straightforward case of greed to me! We let him keep his twenty grand for serving on Big Blue's board. He pockets whatever he gets paid for the patient information he pushes out the door. But that's not enough to satisfy him. He has to open a little pharmacy of his own. What's so confusing about that? And to think I gave that scumbag stock in this organization!"

Peter nervously scratched his head. "No. That's what's confusing. Given what he must be making, there isn't enough missing to make it worth his time or the risks involved in selling it." Then, almost as an afterthought, Peter said, "No. Damien's more likely to be a user himself and a pretty sophisticated one at that."

In the silence that followed this last bombshell, Joshua found himself flashing on his recent mood swings. He'd find something new to level them out.

The intercom buzzed insistently.

"What is it, Mary? You know I'm busy, "Joshua snapped.

"Sorry, Dr. Caliban. It's Mr. Carter again. He says it's urgent, or I wouldn't have bothered you."

"I don't have to tell you how to do your job. You know what to tell him."

"Certainly, Dr. Caliban. What would you like me to tell the O.R.? They've called three times to find out where you are."

Joshua looked over to the clock on his desk. They'd been going at it for almost an hour and a half and he had been due back in surgery at one o'clock.

"Tell them I'll be right over. And Mary, I'm sorry for being so sharp with you. It's all Peter's fault. He has a way of ruining a lunch hour."

Joshua pushed the intercom button off and turned to Peter. "Let's go see if we can save a few lives this afternoon. I'll drop in on Damien before I go home and get his side of the story, if I don't kill him first. You'll need to brief Ross and Roger. And for God's sake, ask them to keep it quiet until we have a better handle on what's going on."

"I'm already scheduled to see them after surgery," Peter said. "Hal is supposed to be getting back to me with some definitive information. We should have a better picture of the damage first thing tomorrow morning."

"Yeah. Presuming we don't hit any more submerged icebergs between now and then. I've still got an urgent meeting with Jane Sherwood before the day is finished."

Joshua noticed Peter wince at his mention of submerged icebergs, start to say something and stop. A sigh escaped his tightened lips.

As they both rose to leave, Joshua caught a glimpse of his face in the mirrored door to his private bathroom. Had he really aged ten years in the last hour and a half?

Thirteen

Although an avowed workaholic, Damien wasn't the kind of man to enjoy a rushed lunch in his office. When he occasionally reached overload, a half-hour walk during the middle of the day helped to clear his mind. But on this particular Monday, he didn't feel like being out in public.

Saturday's retreat had cost him valuable time. This morning the pile on his desk was bigger than usual. Damien's mind was tired, too. Most of the doctors had spent the better part of Saturday berating him in subtle and not-so-subtle ways.

Motor-mouth MacDonald had the finesse of a wounded bull in a china shop. His whining about Elaine getting on his case was pathetic. Talk about pussy whipped! Joshua's tongue-in-cheek suggestion that Peter's investing experience might be of help was insulting. Even Paul had chimed in a few times. Damien had been livid, until Paul explained afterwards that he didn't want to raise any suspicions among the board members about their "special" relationship.

The ungrateful bastards had grabbed onto the salary cut like hungry barracudas and completely ignored the fact that Damien had saved their precious retirement contributions. Totally frustrated, Damien had been goaded into an offensive position. He accused them of having no gratitude, which stirred up such a hornet's nest that he had to backtrack and apologize. Apology didn't come easy for Damien, but in retrospect, the price of eating that small piece of crow was worth the upset he'd caused the vultures.

He knew that the poison rising into his throat again and again was choking him. But how in the hell a bunch of doctors thought they could do a better job running the place was something he'd never fathom. Give them a little management responsibility and they act like experts; let them take a cursory course in finances, and they thought they were little Alan Greenspans. How would they feel if he took an anatomy course and then offered them advice on setting bones? They were so unbelievably arrogant!

All that talk at Friday night's session about managing the organization as if it were a patient was a mixed blessing. Scott MacDonald became even more of a pain in the ass. His chest puffed up with pride when Moerae said health care organizations couldn't achieve excellence unless both the physicians and non-physicians became true win-win partners. As if Scott MacDonald had ever once made an effort to understand Damien's point of view. Jane and Mary had loved that one too. Women always got hooked on the romance of partnerships.

He thought at the time that if Paul could put all those turkeys to sleep, he could indeed get on with the operation. Damien didn't feel threatened by Moerae, at least not in a familiar way. He'd relaxed his guard when she first freely admitted complete ignorance about computers. If he knew where a person was coming from, he could control where they went. And Dr. Moerae King was coming from a backward time as far as technology was concerned. He could skate doughnuts around her. His shoulders loosened and his throat relaxed. With computers on his side, he was unbeatable.

He munched on a tuna sandwich from his favorite deli. They made it with sour cream, not mayonnaise—a small pleasure that salved his anger. Damien worked well under pressure. He aced many exams in college because answers just seemed to present themselves in the heat of the moment. Similarly, the answer to his current predicament had appeared before his eyes while looking over the financial situation on his home computer on Sunday.

It was a brilliant diversionary tactic—at least *he* thought so. Looking at the mounting receivables at C.C.A., Damien was struck with how business had been really picking up. If he could persuade Ashton to make a mid-year adjustment in Big Blue's reimbursement rate to C.C.A., Damien could earn a lot of points with the board. Sure, it would cost Big Blue a few bucks in unearned interest on the float, but that was chump change compared to the eventual payoff.

Fighting through Ashton's resistance when he'd called had been tough, but it had been well worth it. Damien could just picture the big slob as he hemmed and hawed and sputtered on the other end of the line. Few things gave him as much pleasure as watching Ashton squirm.

"I thought we'd agreed at lunch the other day, hypothetically of course, that it was more prudent to avoid wide variations and remain conservative in situations like these," Ashton said.

"What do you suppose would happen if the board sniffed even a hint of a conflict of interest? I think you'll agree that taking this tack serves *both* of our best interests. The adjustment for the end of this year looks like it'll be quite large, and therefore very visible to our auditors."

Ashton finally sighed with resignation. "All right—what do you want me to do?"

"Be a hero. Call Joshua this morning. Congratulate him on the incredible job he must be doing to get his billings to Big Blue so quickly. If he asks any questions about it, just tell him that you were looking over your own reports and you noticed a marked increase in monthly reimbursements to C.C.A. If you can, add in that it's particularly impressive compared to some of the other shops in town."

Ashton loved the strategy. He kept mentioning the chance to make points with higher-ups.

Damien was counting on Joshua being pleased to get the call because, naturally, he'd have been studying the financial information Damien had given him very carefully. All Damien needed to do was make Joshua believe Ashton's change of heart was Damien's doing. Securing the retirement contributions this year was worth points with the docs.

Damien knew Joshua's M.O. pretty well. After a heavy morning of surgery, Joshua would spend the lunch hour in his office. He'd get Ashton's phone message. If Ashton had followed orders about saying he had good news, Mary would be sure that his pink message slip was near the top of the pile.

The intercom buzzed loudly. "Dr. Caliban's office just called."

"I'll take it," he said, straightening quickly.

"I'm sorry, Mr. Rees. Dr. Caliban is not on the line. It was Mrs. Howard who called. Dr. Caliban asked that you not go home today until you hear from him."

"Did she say anything else?"

"No, Mr. Rees. Just that he'd contact you personally before you went home."

Afternoon surgeries would finish no earlier than 4 o'clock. Damien scanned the schedule on his computer. "Would you reschedule my last appointment this afternoon for any time tomorrow? Buzz me the instant you hear from Dr. Caliban and hold all other calls for the rest of the afternoon. I've got some things I have to get done before he calls."

Working feverishly, Damien set about pulling together his data for Joshua, beginning with the spreadsheets. The work went smoothly and quickly, spurred on by his anticipation of Joshua's pleased reception of the job.

❧

Joshua had checked in at his own office before coming over to Damien's, mostly to see if Mary had heard anything more from Jane. She hadn't. He left instructions to interrupt his meeting with Damien the minute Jane's call came through.

What kind of strategy should he adopt with Damien? By playing it cool, maybe he could trap Damien into making an admission without having to force it. But no, Damien was too clever, and Joshua was feeling off-balance. Not only was he still angry, but Peter's discovery of the drug destruction forms brought a feeling of panic to just below the surface. At the very least, to be safe, he'd have to find a temporary way to get his "babies" until the dust settled. At the worst, he'd have to replace Damien as well.

The only way to play it was to go on the offensive immediately. If he concentrated only on the first two transgressions—namely Damien's questionable accounting scheme with Big Blue and his selling of patient records—Damien would be forced to resign. Joshua could figure out a way to do it so Damien could save face. A quiet buyout would avert a lot of very bad publicity. At the same time, many of his medical colleagues outside the board would hail the move as being long overdue. If he were smooth enough, he could convince Peter that the drug destruction problem would disappear along with Damien.

Joshua wrestled only briefly with his own duplicity in the drug matter. Surely he was doing the right thing. How he kept himself going was no one's business, only that he did. He was still on top of the situation. No cause for panic. Besides, C.C.A. would survive Damien's departure—he wasn't so sure about what would happen to his dream-child if he himself were deposed.

By the time he reached Damien's office, Joshua's resolve was so hardened he wore it like a mask over his face. He stood silently at Damien's door. When Damien looked up and Joshua saw Damien's half-smile turn to chagrin, Joshua turned his head and looked back out into the outer office. "No interruptions, except for my secretary."

"Your frat brothers must be giving you a real hazing about the pay cut. You look like a cow whose tits have been pulled through the wringer," Damien started off with forced amiability.

Making sure that the office door was shut, Joshua walked slowly to Damien's desk. He placed his massive hands on the front edge and leaned forward so that his face was directly in front of Damien's. His eyes searched every inch of Damien's face, slowly scanning right to left, up and down. When he'd honed in to exact center and locked his gaze in place, he released his torpedo.

"This is not about a pay cut. It's about behavior that reflects poor judgment. It's about decisions which clearly could be seen as unethical and might even be deemed by a court of law to be illegal. This is about being trusted as a watchdog and shitting on the very people you were supposed to be guarding."

Damien jerked back into his seat, ramming his skull into the cushioned headrest. Rising deliberately from his chair, he leaned across his desk. Like two stags about to bang horns in a battle for territorial rights, they stared at each other silently.

"What the hell has gotten into you, Joshua? You come storming in here, hell bent for leather, like someone's stuck a red-hot poker up your ass. Then, without any explanation whatsoever, you proceed to shit all over me. What are you talking about?"

A thin sneer of a smile crossed Joshua's lip. Damien sneered back, refusing to break the lock Joshua had on his eyes. Joshua didn't really expect Damien to cave in at the first salvo. He would have been disappointed if he had.

"Okay, Damie, let's start with the easy one first," Joshua said with no affection. "Sit down."

Damien complied. Joshua reached across his desk and picked up the telephone. He dialed a number rapidly, pressed the hands-free button, and replaced the receiver.

"Good afternoon. Mr. Simon's office."

"This is Dr. Caliban," Joshua said, glancing at Damien's increasingly flushed face. "Ashton is expecting my call. Is he free at the moment?"

"Certainly, Dr. Caliban. I'll put you right through."

The speakerphone had a way of making people's voices sound hollow and tinny. In Ashton's case, it only accentuated what was already the case.

"Hello, Joshua. How's my favorite butcher? Have I got some good news for you, my friend."

"Save it, Ashton. You're not my friend. And as for the butcher part, I'd never waste my time cutting through your blubber. The good news, I'm pleased to say, is that I have some bad news for you."

The noise from Ashton's end sounded like a horse whinnying. "Close your mouth, Ashton," Joshua said, "unless you've added flies to your diet. I'm going to give you the bottom line and I'm only going to say it once. So listen up good. Effective immediately, Damien has resigned as a member of your board. When you make the announcement, the reason you can give is that he has more pressing duties elsewhere. And be damned sure to praise his contributions."

"Why didn't Damien call me himself?" Ashton barked.

Damien leaned into the phone before Joshua could stop him. "We're on the speakerphone in my office. Shut up and listen."

"That was only half the bad news, Ashton. The really *good* bad news is this: Before the close of business this week, you will deliver to C.C.A. a check in the full amount of the interest you have made on our behalf by investing the float shortfall over the past ten years. I'm sure a man of your business acumen can find an explanation if anyone asks. When I have that check in hand—better yet, after it clears the bank—we can talk about the conditions under which we'll continue to do business."

"That's preposterous!" Ashton sputtered. "Absolutely impossible!"

"That check is in my hand by the end of the day Friday, Ashton, or the next voice you hear will be that of our attorney, Jane Sherwood. She is nowhere near as polite as I am." Joshua hung up the phone and looked to Damien.

When Damien turned away and cleared his throat instead of locking eyes again, Joshua breathed a sigh of relief. Damien had abandoned Ashton. He knew when to cut his own losses.

"That was uncalled for," Damien said, swallowing hard.

Joshua released his grip on the desk and stood up. He locked his fingers and cracked his knuckles. "Oh, really? How so?"

"You and the board were fully supportive of my taking that position on their board when it came up. If you've changed your minds about it being a conflict of interest, you should've said something."

"The only interest-conflict I'm talking about, Damien, has to do with who gets the interest on the float."

"Come on, Joshua. You know better than that. Everybody tries to make some money on the float. We do it ourselves every Friday because people can't get to the bank to cash their checks until Monday."

Joshua was getting tired of the game and knew he had an even tougher issue to raise. "You know goddamn well I'm not talking about month-to-month variations and adjustments," he replied, raising his voice. "I'm talking about year-to-year cumulative shortfalls! Where C.C.A. is always sucking hind tit! And if that's news to you, then I should fire you right on the spot for gross incompetence. Are we done playing games with this one?"

Damien looked unwaveringly back at Joshua. Joshua smiled and flexed his shoulders. Even a hard fighting trout knows when to roll over and quit.

"I will assume," he continued, "until I have information to the contrary, that the only money you made out of the deal was the twenty grand a year we agreed to let you keep as your director's fee. Money, I needn't remind you, that would've been returned to the corporation had you been given the equal treatment with the doctors you always complain is lacking."

For the second time Damien rose. "I know the responsibilities of a board member. That was totally uncalled for."

Damien was obviously feeling the heat to have been baited so easily. But his reaction removed the last hope Joshua had of finding a rational explanation of his second and final issue.

He gripped the desk again and directed his speech at Damien's Adam's apple, which seemed curiously exposed. "You may know the responsibilities of being a board member, but you seem very confused as to the proprietary nature of patient records." Another almost imperceptible swallow moved down Damien's throat. "What in the hell are you talking about? I worked myself to the bone trying to convince you and your money-hungry buddies that we needed the new patient records system. You fought me tooth and nail. Now when people come from around the world to admire the speed and efficiency with which we can transport records, you crow like a rooster in the henhouse. There's no way to win with you guys, Joshua."

Joshua loved the prosecuting attorney role—especially when he had an airtight case. "Peter has hired this computer hack to work with him on the financial review committee I set up. You know Peter is about as much of a computer expert as I am. Anyway, this techno-geek stumbled across the fact that you regularly transfer patient records to the terminal in your office."

"Of course I do, Joshua. I need them to handle the flood of patient complaints that come across this desk every week."

"You requested the Wong file. Did Mr. Wong have a complaint or something? Poor man, he was really shaken."

"*You* asked me to take a look at the file. *You* wanted me to see if I could shave their bill. I did. Which doesn't help reduce the heat we're getting from the docs, by the way. What's the problem?" Damien asked.

Joshua paused. Was Damien genuinely confused? Was he dissembling? Joshua quickly dismissed the thought that Damien might actually think this was about Joshua's grief over the loss of a patient he'd previously saved.

"The problem is, I'm not talking about the file you requested after she died," Joshua spat. "I'm talking about the file you requested two years ago after we almost lost her on the table. I'm talking about selling information to some scumbag company that discounts life insurance policies to families in need, families whose loved ones are terminally ill."

Damien bit his lip to stop its quivering. He pinched his nostrils together and pulled on the hairs in his nose. "I've given my life to building this organization Joshua. And remember, it's your dream, not mine. I know you've wanted to get rid of me for years. This is the last straw. I see no way I can continue. I've taken all the abuse from you and your colleagues I'm going to. You can have my resignation any time you want it."

Joshua slammed his fist down, bouncing the phone off the desk. "You ungrateful son of a bitch! If it wasn't for me, you'd have been out of here a long time ago."

"Fuck, I would have! You're full of shit! Nobody has to take care of me. I take care of myself!"

Joshua reached into his attaché case, flinging the infamous memo onto Damien's desk. "Then you tell me how it is you're still sitting in that chair."

"Shit!" Damien exclaimed as he read it. "I can't believe this. It's impossible … "

The private phone rang, startling them both. "That'll be Mary," Joshua said. "I told her to interrupt me if a certain call came in." He picked up the receiver and nodded. "I'll be right there, Mary. And call Ruth's office. Please tell her not to hold dinner for me. I'll call and let her know later when I expect to be home."

Replacing the receiver, Joshua turned to Damien. "Peter's computer guy has some more digging to do. If his results confirm what I'm sorry to say I believe to be true, I'll have no choice but to ask for your resignation. If we can figure out a way to get back the money you've made from the insurance gig and use it for the benefit of future patients, I may, and I emphasize *may*, be able to prevail upon the board not to institute legal proceedings. For the time being, I want you to take the rest of the week off. I'll call you at home when I've put the rest of the pieces together."

Damien sat silently stunned.

"I'm sorry, Damien," Joshua said, as he walked toward the door.

Damien barely heard him. "Yeah," he said. His jaws ached from gritting his teeth, his voice barely a whisper.

Fourteen

Paul Blake moved his hand inch by inch over the front of Elaine's bikini underwear, enjoying the exquisite magnetic tension between his fingers and the silky white satin. The hairs on his hand stood at attention and the lightning fingers flashing across the Chicago skyline illuminated the blackness of the hair springing out from beneath the elastic edges. Coarse, thick hair that cushioned the magnificent bulge of his genitals bunched under the stretched crotch of the panties. He loved wearing them, touching them, looking at himself in them. The contrast between the fabric, so lusciously female, and his skin, so deliciously male—and *forbidden*, delighted him nearly to the point of sexual release.

Since childhood, Paul had loved the tension teasing brought. He especially enjoyed playing with magnetic tension. He would hold two large magnets, one in each hand, the prongs pointing toward each other. The challenge was to see how long he could postpone the magnets' final joining, slowly allowing them to draw closer and closer together as smoothly as possible in increments of centimeters until the prongs met with a dull clink.

There were rules. For example, his hands had to move simultaneously. As the gap between the magnets narrowed, the force of attraction between the opposite poles increased. He would tease himself, pulling his hands back just enough to keep the magnets apart. Then he'd gradually allow them another inch closer. Naturally, the closer the poles came to connecting, the more concentration he had to exercise.

After a while, his hands would begin to twitch as they were doing now. His mind would begin to chatter. Why don't we stop this silly game? Let's get on with it, get to the climax. You can do it again. It will be slower the second time around.

He learned how to resist these thoughts, because the climax of any game wasn't nearly as interesting as the process. The play that set up the shot that always engaged him more than the ultimate goal.

He thought lazily of Scott MacDonald as he continued to stroke himself. Now there was a man whose understanding of foreplay was definitely unimaginative. Would it have something to do with golf? No? No wonder he had found it pathetically easy to usurp Scott's rightful place in his wife's bed, not to mention the forbidden territories deep inside her.

Paul let his hand stray up to rest on one of Elaine's pendulous breasts. They were truly a structural marvel. He needed three fingers including his thumb to massage her nipple. When erect, it was bigger than some cocks he'd sucked as a kid. She'd told him one day that they were bigger than some she'd sucked, too. Then she did a most extraordinary thing: She gathered up her massive breasts, one at a time, to her own lips and started licking and sucking the nipples herself. It drove him crazy.

That was the great thing about Elaine. She'd do almost anything when it came to sex. But best of all, Paul loved to sit on her chest facing her and watch her suck the tip of his cock while he squeezed it between her massive tits. When her nipples turned rosy pink and stood up straining to be kissed, he'd raise himself up to squat over her face. She'd lick his balls while he came.

A rush of heat flooded his neck and face. He rolled over slightly to take the swollen tip of her breast into his mouth.

Elaine moaned deeply. "Oh, I like this. I like this a lot."

"Oh, yeah?" he said, without removing his lips. "What do you like about it?"

"I love feeling your cock when it's rubbing up against the inside of my panties. I love seeing the little wet spot you make."

"A sign of things to *come*," he whispered.

Elaine pushed her other breast up against the one he was sucking. "This one's feeling left out."

He didn't stop immediately, so Elaine pushed harder. He circled her nipple with his tongue, rolling it in his mouth, and sucked harder until he finally allowed it to be gently tugged out. Elaine rewarded him with a long, low moan.

"Okay, what else do you really like?"

"Hmmm." She thrust her breast against his face. "Let me see. This is hard." She reached down to caress him. "What I love, what I really love, is when you pull the backside of my panties together, so that they're hidden tight in the crack. That drives me wild. You have no idea how gorgeous your ass looks like that."

His hands slid down off her breasts. "Your wish is my command. And when you get wild, what do you want to do?"

Elaine licked her lips like a cat. She slid down the length of his body until her ear was covering his belly button, while her hands slithered over his groin. She curled several fingers around the elastic waistband of her panties, there in the space where his straining cock had pulled the flimsy fabric away from his stomach.

"And then, I would rip them off of you like this!" She squealed like a kid tearing the wrapping off a Christmas present. Three urgent tugs and her underwear hung shredded from Paul's waist. "And I'd eat whatever I found wrapped inside."

As Elaine began to suck in earnest, Paul let his mind wander to keep the tension up longer. What a way to do business. Elaine was one of the key players in Paul's scheme to wreak vengeance on Joshua Caliban. Lucky she was so sexually needy and so open to kinky exploration of her desires. Paul's plan was satisfying in its baroque complexities. Each piece of the whole required exquisite manipulation in order to complement every other piece.

Take Damien, for instance. Removing Damien from power was only a stepping stone to ousting Joshua as head of C.C.A. Guilt—at least a little guilt—tweaked him for using Damien that way, but after all, all was fair in love and war. Those pesky attacks of conscience rarely lasted anyway. In fact, they disappeared as quickly as the periodic payments Damien gave him from their Care, Inc. scam.

Paul could not have asked for a better response from Joshua than his unwillingness to get rid of Damien, because it had turned the doctors away from their CEO. And Paul kept the docs' discontent potent by inciting Scott to fan the flames of suspicion among the board members. He controlled Scott through Elaine. And Elaine, well, he controlled Elaine through her insatiable appetite for sexual variety.

Paul suggested ways for Elaine to "sympathize" with her husband over the trials and tribulations he had to endure at C.C.A. She enjoyed alternating this tender approach with demands for new and more exciting things she and Scott could do in bed. A pussy whipped puppy dog trained to capitulate to her every lust. It amused Paul to imagine how poor Scott suffered perpetually from performance anxiety.

For her part, Elaine insisted that she hated Scott's slobbering all over her. When she complained, Paul would always remind her that one day they'd be rid of Scott. He dangled the idea of marriage in front of her until she became insistent about a time line, then he'd jerk the notion away like a ball on a rubber string.

Elaine was trying to tell him something. "Your burber, your burber," she said around a mouthful of cock. What? Oh! His beeper was ringing.

"Keep going! I'm coming!" He grabbed her head and thrust his hips in time with her bobbing.

"Almost coitus interruptus," she said smiled slyly while diligently licking the last few drops oozing from the tip of his cock.

He reached across to turn off the pager. "Almost only counts in horseshoes." His tone turned cooler—almost dismissive, "That thunderstorm will really snarl traffic. You'll need a little extra time to get home. You've got some pretty important work to do tonight."

Elaine dutifully got out of the bed, paused to stretch languidly, presenting her full cheeks to Paul as she arched backwards, then headed for the bathroom. She grabbed a spare pair of panties from her bag on the way.

"All right. But first, a quick shower and I'm out of here. And don't think for a red-hot minute I'm looking forward to trying to influence Scott tonight," she said pouting.

"You'll do your job and you'll like it, or I'll smack your bottom," Paul said, winking.

The number flashing on his beeper was Damien's private line. Paul swore under his breath. Damien knew this was Paul's afternoon off. If his call weren't urgent, he'd have left a message on Paul's answering machine instead of paging him. Shit.

⁂

Damien furiously smashed the phone back onto its cradle. No way Paul was playing a round of golf in this weather. No, more likely he's gripped in the sweaty embrace of one of his honeys.

His head was still spinning, even though Joshua had been gone for twenty minutes. His shock was so profound, he couldn't identify his feelings, let alone sort them out. Had he actually been that stupid? To be duped by the very person he'd allowed to come within shouting distance emotionally? Being stupid was more infuriating than being betrayed. More frightening than to admit that another human being was fallible was the discovery that he could lose control of a single facet of his life.

Paul had some explaining to do. Even if he had a good answer, the two of them still had a heap of trouble on their hands. The issue of the Big Blue directorship was no big deal by itself. At the worst, Damien anticipated getting his hands slapped. If he could calm Joshua down, it might even turn out to be a plus. He'd get a lot of mileage with the docs from a sudden cash windfall. Damien hated to admit it, but Joshua's handling of Ashton Simons on the phone was a work of art. Ashton must have been shitting in his pants.

But the discovery of the insurance scam was a serious upset. Of course, it couldn't last forever, but he would have preferred it to end on his own terms, not Joshua's. Self-doubt was an entirely new factor to consider—one with which Damien was not familiar. How good was this hack of Peter's? Surely not up to his own level. What kind of threat did this Hal Mays really present?

Time for a contingency plan. He drummed his fingers on the mouse pad. The worst-case scenario would entail the return of all the money he'd made from Big Blue to C.C.A. It was out of the question. Even if he were able to parachute into the safety of Big Blue on a permanent basis, he'd want that insurance money as his nest egg. It was safely tucked away in an offshore bank. No reason to panic.

The second scenario, which wasn't much better, would require that he figure out a way to lay his hands on a new chunk of cash. Joshua would do everything in his power to prevent Damien going to prison. C.C.A. couldn't stand the publicity, and Joshua's ego couldn't stand the deflation. They'd cut a deal, that much was certain. What wasn't clear was how much he'd have to forfeit.

The second the red light flashed on his private line, Damien grabbed the receiver.

"What in the hell are you doing paging me in the middle of my afternoon off?" Paul barked.

Damien smiled bitterly. Good old Paul. When in doubt, attack. "What's the matter, Paul baby? Did I catch you in midstream? I'll tell you what I'm doing. I'm trying to track down a snake in the grass so I can shove a red-hot poker up his ass."

"What are you talking about? I was just working on Elaine MacDonald. This is a delicate situation, which I'm not sure you fully appreciate. Elaine is critical in the handling of her dear husband, Scottie-boy. She's got to get him to increase the pressure on Joshua."

Damien swiveled his middle finger in the air. "I'll bet you were working real hard on her."

"Jesus Christ, Damien. Is this jealousy raising its ugly head again? We've been over this before. You know how important she is to our plan."

"Yeah, but I thought our plan was to find a way to get rid of Joshua!" Damien replied. "You'd better have a damn good explanation as to why Joshua received an ultimatum from a portion of the board, dated June first, demanding my removal. You've been double-crossing me, Paul, and I'm going to get even."

Hearing Damien's direct threat, Paul had to use brute force to quell the angry answer rising in his throat; instead, he replied evenly, "Don't get your balls in an uproar, sweetie. You've got to calm down in order to make sense."

Damien clenched his fist and gritted his teeth. "Don't give me that placating sweetie shit. Our great plan is in big trouble.

Joshua wouldn't have shown me that memo unless all hell had broken loose in the organization."

"I'm not placating you, asshole. I just don't want you going off half-cocked. Our plan hasn't changed one iota," Paul said. "In fact, if you'll shut up and listen for a minute, I'll tell you how it's gotten stronger."

"I'm all ears."

"The point—let's remember the point—is that we want to get rid of Joshua, right? Well, I could tell from talking with guys like Ross and Roger that a direct assault on Joshua wasn't going to work. I found out they think *you're* the problem. They have absolutely no idea that without you, this place would go to hell in a handbasket."

Damien smiled and relaxed his fist. The power behind the throne might one day still wear the crown. "And don't you forget it."

"Through Elaine's intervention," Paul went on, "I had Scott plant the seed in Ross's ears, in Roger's, and some of the other's, that Joshua was getting fed up with your inability to get the doctors off his back. The pay cut was the last straw. After that, it was real easy to convince Ross and Roger that we were just doing our jobs as board members to draft that memo on Joshua's behalf."

"Yeah, but … "

"Hold your tongue a few more seconds, will you, please? I know you're upset, but you're beating the wrong horse."

"Okay, okay. But get on with it," Damien said, trying to mask his disbelief.

"Joshua may be the only other person besides me who knows how good you really are. After all, he was the one who brought you into the organization, wasn't he? So I knew there was no way he'd react positively to that memo. In fact, it was spectacular. He was so pissed. When he got that memo, he totally lost his cool. Now, there are a lot of people wondering about his judgment. So you see, he helped us by his reaction. By under-mining his own credibility, he actually made our job easier."

"I doubt that, and I'll tell you why in a minute. But first you tell me why you didn't let me know about this before. Joshua had me by the balls this afternoon."

"I never imagined Joshua would show you the memo. But think about it. The fact that Joshua knew he'd caught you by the short hairs today guarantees that he has no idea that you're in bed with anyone on the board. Even if he had the slightest sus-picion, he'd probably assume it'd be motor-mouth MacDonald. He'd never guess it was me in a million years. As for me, I was saving the memo for you myself as a gift for the celebration party you and I are going to have soon."

Damien's brow curled as he examined Paul's explanation with every analytical cell in his brain. "The chances of my becoming president," he said, "took a severe nosedive today. Joshua ran all over me in my own office this afternoon. I'm telling you, he reamed my ass out."

"He's done it to me too, remember. But we've been through tough times before and came out smelling like roses. We'll do it this time too. The important thing is to stay cool."

"Easier for you to say than for me to do," Damien replied.

"Listen, Damien. Trust me. Nothing's going to happen imme-diately and you're not in this alone. It'll take Joshua a few days to sort everything out. He told you that himself."

Damien ran his finger over the scar on his chin and sighed. "Yeah. He even told me to take a few days off and not come into the office."

"Great! That'll give me time to nose around tomorrow and see what's really going down. And it'll free you up to find a loop-hole."

"I hope the loophole doesn't turn out to be a noose around my neck. Make that *our* necks."

"Don't threaten me, Damien." Paul sounded like a cornered attack dog.

Damien smiled and rubbed his nose. Another assault. "Just a reminder, Paul. Just a reminder."

"Okay. I'll give you a call tomorrow," Paul said. "We'll get together in the evening. I'd come over tonight, but Elaine sucked me dry and you've had enough frustration for one day. Meanwhile, think positive. It's amazing what can happen overnight."

"Bring a little 'something extra' with you tomorrow. By then, I'll need it."

"You got it. Something you'll never forget. Gotta run," Paul said.

Damien hung up the phone. Something in Paul's tone bothered him, but he couldn't place it so he dismissed it and stepped to a set of file drawers that walled his office. While listening to Paul, he'd remembered one of his past brilliant ideas. He had come up with a way to repay C.C.A. and simultaneously take out some insurance in case the whole Care, Inc. scam came to light. He grabbed a blank set of patient record forms, stuffed several into his attaché case, and switched on the modem connected to his computer. He had a lot of work to do from home tonight.

⁓ঔৣ⁓

Hal Mays sat glued to a pair of flashing screens. This was just the kind of job he loved to take on. He'd gotten a reputation for brilliance in the uses and abuses of computer technology. Even the IRS had employed him to instruct their investigators. But what really sold clients was his straight-arrow ethics.

Hal's "hippie" looks ran more than skin deep. Raging greed really bugged him. To his mind, it had caused the present condition of the earth, with its ozone depletion and damaged rainforests. Values lost to profits every time. Sure, the world was full of gradations of color and shades of gray. But as far as values were concerned, a person was either good or bad. Hal didn't aspire to heroism, but he felt this job offered him an easy chance to do something good.

He'd known from the outset that Dr. Peter Albert was a good guy. Most doctors Hal knew were a lot of stuffed shirt Harvard MBA-types who wouldn't give the time of day to a sandal-shod guy with long gray braided hair and a pointed beard. But Peter had been respectful and appreciative of Hal's skills immediately. And he'd also surmised that what Peter needed to know concerned more than a routine checkup of C.C.A.'s internal systems.

Yesterday morning, Hal had Peter show him what kind of equipment Damien had in his office. Hal noted the special modem on Damien's machine. Bingo. Just now, the light flashing on Hal's screen told him that the modem had been switched on. If he was patient—and he was a patient man—he could determine when another modem someplace else called the one in Damien's office. He prayed that he'd be lucky enough to have time to determine its source.

Hal had already worked out some of the logistics of C.C.A.'s internal system. The trolls installed to protect the system from invasion had recorded the sources and dates of several such incidents. In particular, the computer in Damien's office had requested to see certain patient records from C.C.A.'s central files.

He scribbled himself a reminder note to research the pharmacy records.

In another few minutes, he'd have the access number to Damien's home computer. Damien would then be an open book, one that Hal could read from his own room, which was an especially pleasant aspect of the job. As another roll of thunder stampeded across the Chicago sky, he thanked the good Lord he wouldn't be out in that storm and rush hour traffic.

As for Damien, the poor bastard, Hal figured it'd take him quite a while to get home. Hal double-checked the address on his notepad. He had enough time to take a piss and make a pot of coffee. This could be a long stakeout.

Fifteen

Jane Sherwood's sleek and contemporary office exuded a quiet elegance and order that implied someone had poured buckets of money into it. It was more a reflection of the innately discerning taste that Jane had cultivated since childhood than mere indulgence. She'd often joked that if she got tired of lawyering she'd become an interior decorator.

The L-shape, floor-to-ceiling glass walls offered a sweeping view of Chicago from skyline to shoreline. The other two walls housed a library full of volumes covering every aspect of law, medicine, and art. The Italian leather couches were deep and comfortable and made to order in Jane's favorite color, deep midnight blue. This was the color of the pineal chakra and hence the symbol of a visionary. The coffee table was a work of art. Two sculpted arms formed its base. As they reached to the heavens, each supported a slab of marble inlaid with silver on its fingers.

Jane turned in her chair to stare at Lake Michigan. Sail boats and wind surfers cut a crisscross pattern through the rolling whitecaps. The sky's dull leaden color heavy with moisture that wouldn't let go seemed to echo her dismal reflections on the retreat the other night.

Everyone had nodded dutifully when Moerae, in her opening remarks, asked if they believed all patients could be healed but not cured. But when she asked how many of them had actually walked up to a colleague and said, "I have concerns about your abilities as a healer," mouths dried up. No one wanted to point a finger for fear that it might get pointed back. The absence of measurable standards of behavior acceptable to the docs left damn little chance of learning from past mistakes. Instead, back-biting and character assassination had become the accepted mode of feedback for most of her clients. Like rats in a maze or gerbils on a wheel, history repeated itself in ugly reruns.

A pile of pending malpractice suits towered on her desk. She frowned. These days, lawyers didn't need to chase ambulances to roust out work. The patients did that on their own, incited by TV advertisements that bloomed with the speed of mushrooms after a heavy rain, poisoning the national consciousness with a driving urge to sue.

More often than not, she didn't see a case until it was almost time to sign on the bottom line, since out-of-court settlements were the objective whenever possible. To further this practice, Illinois, as had many other states, instituted a mandatory mal-practice review board. These review boards were small groups made up of health care providers, lawyers, and, occasionally, laypersons. They were presided over by a judge. The function of the review board would be to act as a screen. It could recom-mend binding arbitration or allow a case to go through the for-mal legal system. Although she supervised all the cases, Jane would only become personally involved in those her staff thought might actually go to court. One of those case files sat on top of the pile in front of her, an ominous looking note clipped to the corner.

Her colleague, Sam Gould, was a really level-headed guy, not prone to histrionics in or out of the courtroom. So he must have had a damn good reason for his note to her, which read, "I can't believe this one will ever see the inside of a court room. But if it does, it will make the old pedicle-screw suit look like kids having a water fight."

The plaintiff's attorney was scheduled to deliver his closing argument to the review board just after lunch. Sam wanted Jane to hear it firsthand. Jane stuffed the report into her leather case. She would have time to study it on her way to the review board office.

Reaching across her desk, she pushed the intercom and had Liz call her a cab—one with working air conditioning, please.

She pressed one of the automatic dialing buttons on her phone, and Moerae's answering machine picked up. "Moerae, this is Jane calling. Sorry, babe, I have to cancel our shopping date this afternoon. Leave some clothes for me, will you?"

In the cool quiet of the taxi, Jane picked up the report Sam had prepared with the background material. An uncomfortable feeling settled into her stomach.

A few moments later, she slumped down. "Damn," she muttered under her breath. This one could get messy. Upon the recommendation of his C.C.A. physician to help curb his

hypertensive type-A personality and reduce the probability of another acute myocardial infarction, Mr. LaPorte had enrolled in C.C.A.'s wellness program. Mr. LaPorte complained several times to the teacher with no effect that the meeting room was too cold, according to his wife.

If Joshua knew that C.C.A. employees were ignoring patient feedback, he'd have a heart attack of his own. Mrs. LaPorte's words struck like a sword: "When I picked him up at the end of the session, he was screaming with rage, shivering from the cold and coughing up tons of phlegm."

Jane shook her head. What were the odds? But odds didn't matter. In today's adversarial health care environment riddled with mutual mistrust between patients and their providers, only the bottom line mattered. In spite of the cold in the taxi, Jane found herself wiping perspiration from her own brow as she turned to the final page of the report, hoping against hope she'd misread it. No. Mr. LaPorte had been pronounced dead on arrival at C.C.A.'s emergency room. Cause of death: a rupture of the myocardium resulting in cardiac tamponade.

Mr. LaPorte, in his frustration and weakened physical state, had blown a gasket and his widow was holding C.C.A. accountable. Jane shuddered.

The cab driver asked, "Too cold for you, ma'am? I can warm it up some."

"No, thanks. I'll be fine. I can see the building just ahead." She reached into her bag for her cell phone, which had begun to beep with an urgent page.

The message was urgent. "Call Dr. Caliban's office ASAP," Liz's voice stated emphatically. If she hadn't been stepping out into an unseasonable Chicago heat wave, Jane might have shuddered again.

She paid the cabbie, eschewing her cell phone for more privacy, ran for the nearest enclosed pay phone. "Mary, it's Jane. What's up?"

"Sorry to bother you, Jane, but I've had a series of unusual calls I thought you should know about."

"Shoot. I'm in a phone booth outside the Medical Malpractice Review Board. I'm late for a hearing."

"Virgil Carter, head of the Bar Association, called this morning for Dr. Caliban. Wanted to get his comments on, quote, 'an interesting new malpractice case we were facing.'"

Jane swallowed hard. "Did he happen to mention the name of the plaintiff?"

"The LaPorte family, I believe."

"Ouch."

"Not five minutes after he calls, the news desk at CBS calls, sniffing around at the same issue."

"Shit." If the plaintiff's attorney was already trying to fire up public pressure, Sam's premonition of imminent trouble was taking on added credence. Lawyers called it *chumming*, which was exactly like whipping up a school of piranhas into a feeding frenzy.

"Listen, Mary, I've got to run. Make sure, make absolutely certain, that everyone follows normal procedure on this one. Could you please tell Liz the same. And tell Joshua I'll see him this afternoon, but it may not be until close to five-thirty. I'll call as soon as I'm done here."

The plaintiff's attorney, Garth Haskins, was beginning his closing argument to the review panel as Jane slid into the seat beside Sam. Sam's weak smile was not encouraging. She closed her eyes briefly and focused on the space between her eyes, grounding herself in that celestial midnight blue color that always conjured up serenity. She'd need every scrap of concentration she could muster. She had so little respect for and nearly loathed Haskins, the senior partner of the firm that promised, 'If we can't win for our clients, we don't take the case." Listening to his egotistical points of view always actively challenged her spiritual aspirations.

If only he weren't so good-looking. In spite of her natural inclinations, she'd always admired his thick, salt-and-pepper hair sleekly styled away from his temples and his handsome Aryan features. He was the picture of a successful, confident, totally correct lawyer. He could have modeled in a Calvin Klein ad. But the picture was flawed. The smirk on his face was fatuous as far as she was concerned. Unfortunately, to the review board listening to his arguments, it probably would only seem to register distaste at the treatment of the deceased.

Haskins was hammering on exactly the points she'd expected. Coldness of the room. People wearing summer clothes. Impossible to relax. LaPorte following his doctor's prescription.

Taking responsibility for his own health and behavior. When Haskins paused in his staccato beat, Jane looked up. A trump card was coming.

"As we've heard in Dr. Miller's expert testimony, here was a man who'd been making a good recovery from his recent heart attack."

Jane looked down at the scribbled note Sam had pushed in front of her. "Miller's a big shot from Mayo," it read.

Jane winced. The heavy hits were coming.

"Dr. Miller has testified that Mr. LaPorte's upper respiratory infection developed into viral pneumonia, which produced an even greater strain on a heart that was already receiving an insufficient supply of oxygen. Add to this Mr. LaPorte's extreme frustration that he couldn't change any of the uncomfortable and ultimately health-threatening conditions in a wellness program, which he felt obligated to attend for the sake of his health. When that portion of the heart wall that was already weakened by the first attack gave out, Mr. LaPorte suffered a fatal heart attack."

Haskins cast a fish-cold eye at Jane's table. Afraid the heat would flash from her eyes, Jane worked to keep her expression neutral. What an insufferable, self-righteous prick the man was.

"C.C.A.'s management weren't ignorant of this situation or its consequences," Haskins continued. "Several other people in the wellness program had complained of stiff necks from the air conditioning and reported upper respiratory ailments as a result of the cold. When they asked for a warmer place to study, many of the patients were treated rudely by hospital staff members. Even the instructors had pleaded for relief from the cold on several documented occasions. They were treated no better. C.C.A.'s repeated response ... " He paused dramatically and thumbed through his notes, grinning from ear to ear. " ... 'Bring sweaters!' was really just another way of saying, 'Let them eat cake.' I ask you, ladies and gentlemen, is that response consistent with any definition of cradle-to-grave quality care?"

Did the attorney have proof for that statement? Jane looked sideways at Sam and raised an eyebrow. He read her question and nodded discreetly. She swallowed hard. The next fusillade of bullets hit the heart of Haskins' case. Premeditated. Full knowledge of the problem. Failure to uphold fiduciary responsibility. Every employee a provider of human warmth and caring.

She quickly scribbled a note to check that point with Moerae, and then pushed back the bile she felt rising in her throat. Haskins was such a hypocrite. What did he know about being warm and caring.

"You have heard defendant's counsel claim that C.C.A.'s management need not be highly skilled medical professionals," Garth Haskins said, a sneer painted across his hatchet face. Hands on hips, he walked slowly towards the table where Jane and Sam were seated. He stopped, pulled a pen from his vest pocket, and pointed it like a sword at Sam Gould's heart. "Mr. Gould has claimed that neither C.C.A.'s method of administering their wellness program nor the doctor had anything whatsoever to do with this specific case."

Haskins returned his gaze to the panel. "Ladies and gentlemen, this is the same as saying that a heart failure wouldn't produce a fatality because the lungs were still perfectly good." Haskins paused to acknowledge the subtle titter that rippled through the jury panel. "The defendant's counsel has further claimed that Dr. Rupman, upon whose recommendation, I remind you, Mr. LaPorte enrolled in the wellness program, could not have known about the cold room, much less have been responsible for it."

Winning the lottery couldn't have brought a rosier glow to Garth Haskins' cheeks. Jane had beaten him badly on a few occasions recently, and he must relish evening the score.

Wiping the smile from his face, Haskins turned to glower at Jane. "There's nothing in either C.C.A.'s advertising campaigns or its definition of quality care that can excuse any of its personnel from performing as the highly skilled professionals they must be. Nothing can excuse any of its personnel from using *all* human and technological means available to heal patients. Failure to live up to that promise, on any employee's part, should result in immediate dismissal. C.C.A. failed to live up to that promise and it cost Mr. LaPorte his life. Let me read you defense counsel's exact words in this regard." He extended his hand to receive the page from the transcribed proceedings his law clerk passed to him.

He had this whole thing scripted down to a T. Jane fought the nausea.

"Mr. Gould's exact words were," Haskins continued, "'C.C.A. is a very complex organization. You'd have to be a god to know every little detail of what goes on.' Only gods would believe that they have no need for a wellness program," Haskins said, twisting the knife. "C.C.A.'s personnel are not gods. They are imperfect human beings like you and me. So where, we need to ask ourselves, do C.C.A.'s own employees go for their wellness training? One possibility is that Dr. Rupman and some of his colleagues choose to participate in a wellness program offered by another hospital."

The members of the review panel squirmed. The layperson and the nurse smiled broadly at that little dig. The overweight lawyer and the doctor stiffened.

Jane sat forward as Haskins proceeded to plant the seeds of reasonable doubt. How could C.C.A.'s doctors recommend their wellness program if they hadn't experienced it themselves? What if they'd never been to any wellness program? Worse yet, what if they had attended C.C.A.'s wellness program and knew of the cold conditions?

Haskins held his palms out and paused to allow those seeds to grab root. He moved to the table and thumbed through his piled up papers, as if checking any points he'd missed. A standard ploy to make certain everyone was watching closely just before delivering the finishing blow.

"Ladies and gentlemen, the issue in this case is not how many, if any, of C.C.A.'s personnel attended their own wellness program. This case is about truth in advertising. It's about organizational integrity. In the vernacular, it's about walking the talk. In this case, Care Corporation of America has made two premeditated promises, wellness and quality care. We must not tolerate, and we must not allow the profession to which we entrust our wellness to tolerate, a single false promise. Thank you for your kind attention."

The judge leaned forward to look at the clock on the office wall. "In view of the late hour and the complicated nature of this case, I wonder if counsel for the defense might not agree to wait until tomorrow to make his closing argument. I don't want to start and be unable to finish."

"The gods are smiling on us," Sam whispered to Jane. "Thank you, your Honor," he said. "My colleague has uncovered some new information, in light of which the defense requests that the panel postpone reconvening until tomorrow afternoon. I'm confident we can wrap this up by then."

The judge's eyebrows curled and she shot a half-smile at Haskins. "If council for the plaintiff has no objections, I see no problem."

Garth Haskins knew better than to object. The panel would appreciate the morning off. Besides, it would give the defense time to mull over the news leak he'd no doubt arranged. "No problem, your Honor," Haskins said.

Jane's anxiety threatened to choke her. She hadn't said anything to Sam about new information. She didn't, in fact, have any. If Sam was bluffing at that high a level, it meant the defense must have a very weak hand.

"This isn't smelling good," she whispered. "You know I have no news at all."

Sam nodded and stuffed his papers into his leather bag. "But *I* do, and it isn't good. Let's get out of here."

As they slid into the back seat of the cab, Jane turned to Sam. "Okay, I have a hunch I'm going to be sorry I asked, but what's the new news?"

"With hunches like yours, I should take you to the track." He paused, rubbed his eyes wearily, the sagging skin around them not quickly snapping back. "My informants at CBS hinted that the whole affair will be featured on the six o'clock news tonight."

Jane grabbed her cellular, feeling sick to her stomach. "Hi, Mary, it's Jane. Please tell Joshua I'm on my way back. I'll see him in his office by five-thirty at the latest. No. It isn't looking too good."

She quickly dialed a second number. "I'm not going to make it home, love. A crisis is breaking loose. I'll be in the office and the law library all night. Tape the six o'clock news for me. I'll call you later." She ignored Sam's surprised look. "I know, I know, I'm being uncharacteristically brusque," she teased, then she sobered. She stared evenly into his blood shot eyes and folded her delicate hands into her lap. "So what do you think, counselor?"

"I'd say there's a big storm blowing up in the Windy City. It's a case we could probably win through attrition, if nothing else," he said. "But I don't believe Haskins will allow us to drag the case out that long. His will to fight is ferocious, as you well know. But I'll tell you, this case could be the tip of an iceberg. When it melts, it could initiate such a flood of similar suits there will be more organizations than ours sinking into the ocean. And I don't just mean in the health care industry."

"Sam, you know what I love about you? Your grasp of the far-reaching significance in any complicated situation. You must have something in mind so give it to me. What do you mean, not 'just health care'?"

Sam turned to Jane and tapped a finger in the palm of his hand. "What they're basically charging is that there's a relationship between the way we manage our staff and the quality of the healing culture patients experience when they come in for care. If we treat our people badly, they'll pass it on to the patients. It's a sort of 'what-goes-around-comes-around' argument."

Jane's head throbbed. What Sam was saying was an echo of Moerae's thinking. "What's that got to do with a non-health care organization?"

Sam yawned and gulped a deep breath. "Think about how many different kinds of organizations affect your life. You can bet the managers of these enterprises can be as cold and indifferent as some of our administrators are, not to mention our doctors. If I were the plaintiff's attorney, I'd be stirring up some class action suits in large corporations as well. Why not take advantage of this notion of managerial malpractice?"

She shook her head, massaging her temples.

"Let's face it, Jane. For most people, the handcuffs they're wearing aren't made of gold. Lots of people feel mistreated by their bosses. And they are! But most employees also feel they have no choice but to take it."

"Thanks, counselor. Got any more exciting possibilities?"

Sam shrugged as he paid the cab driver. "Hey, you asked me for my opinion."

"Yeah. And you know I value it. I was looking for some good news to bring Joshua. It doesn't sound like the six o'clock broadcast will give it to him."

"It's getting to be a crazy world, Jane. Want me to stay to help later tonight?"

"I'd really appreciate that. Thanks."

"No sweat. That's the least I can do when my boss is willing to sacrifice a hot date herself." He grinned at her. "Good luck with the boss. I'll see you later."

Riding the elevator to Joshua's office, she tried desperately to visualize any number of optimistic outcomes. She failed completely.

"Hi, Mary. Is Joshua in there?" she asked, nodding toward his closed door.

"He just came storming back from Damien's office ten minutes ago. Growled at me like a treed lion. Slammed his door so hard, it felt like an earthquake." A vertical line etched between her brows.

"Well, hold on to your seat. I might send him over eight on the Richter scale."

"I took the liberty of pulling together some papers I thought you might need for your meeting," Mary said.

The label on the file, LAPORTE: CONFIDENTIAL, was newly typed. "God bless you, darlin'. You're an unsung hero. Let him know I'm here, will you?" Mary smiled brightly.

"Dr. Caliban, Ms. Sherwood is here," Mary said formally, and then stiffened.

"Great. Send her right in. And, Mary … uh, sorry, really sorry, about snapping at you."

The two women looked at each other in dismay.

"It sounds like the roaring lion has been transformed into a sweet pussy cat!" Jane said in a stage whisper. "What in the world do you think he's on?"

Mary's hand flew up to cover her gaping mouth and a forced smile took its place. "What can I tell you? Just like the Chicago weather. If you don't like it, wait a minute and it'll change."

Joshua's relaxed smile caught Jane off guard when she first walked into his office, but her ease dissolved when he cut straight to the chase.

"I gather there's a great white swimming around in our waters. How big is it?"

Jane glanced at her watch. Almost twenty minutes before the news went on. "Could be messy. Nothing definite yet. It sounds like you didn't have the kind of day to write home about. What's up with Damien? Mary said you looked fit to be tied after your meeting with him."

He shifted. So he hadn't made up his mind how much to tell her.

In a voice as cold as a steel scalpel he said, "It looks like I'll have to ask for Damien's resignation."

In preparation for courtroom depositions, Jane had coached Joshua many times in the strategy of answering the question asked exactly and giving nothing else. How irritating to have him pull it on her.

"Come on, Joshua, we don't have time for courtroom games. This is me you're talking to. What in the name of Christ does that mean?"

Joshua delivered a thorough, ten-minute summary of the Damien situation in the same matter-of-fact tone, as though he was talking about a total stranger rather than someone he'd worked with and stood by for years. Dumping all attachment to a man the second he was out the door didn't compute, but it didn't seem worth arguing at the moment.

"How soon?" she asked curtly, adopting his style.

"As soon as Peter pulls together all the computer records. Take a look at Damien's contract tomorrow and let me know what the complications might be. For the time being, I've told Damien to take some vacation time."

215

"Give me a second. Mary just gave me this file." She scanned the file's contents, not looking up until she was finished.

"Are they serious, or is this another legal holdup?" Joshua asked.

She went to the TV set built into the wall of Joshua's office. "I think we're-about to find out."

"And now for some local news," the anchorwoman said. "The charges in a recent malpractice suit have stunned the medical profession. Although some claim to have foreseen such a case coming for years, few were prepared for the nature of the charges, which the survivors of prominent restaurateur J.P. LaPorte brought against his physician, Dr. E.B. Rupman and Care Corporation of America.

"In an exclusive interview with CBS News, the plaintiff's attorney, Garth Haskins, said he intends to prove that LaPorte's death was the direct result of false advertising and the managerial malpractice of quality care, not the management of his technical care but the management of the organization responsible for providing his care. By focusing on issues the legal system has not previously considered in medical malpractice suits, Mr. Haskins noted, this case could set a precedent."

Joshua stared at the screen intently, and Jane groaned as Haskins' image floated onto the screen. He was walking out of the review. She saw herself in the background, blurred and indistinct, still inside the judge's office. The reporter continued: "'The real problem,' he told CBS, 'is that many health care organizations fail to deliver what they must, regardless of whether or not they advertise explicitly.' He is confident that the Medical Malpractice Review Board will agree with his conclusion that, 'We must not tolerate, and we must not allow the profession to which we entrust our wellness to tolerate, a single false promise.' Officials from C.C.A. were unavailable for comment."

The announcer turned to her broadcasting partner. "Well, Jim, the next time your blood pressure goes up because your doctor kept you waiting for an hour, you may have recourse for the disease you incurred. When we return, we'll bring you some more familiar local disease as the Cubs dropped two to the Cardinals."

Jane rubbed her neck. The segue from the malpractice case to the local sports disappointment appalled her.

"This one could really get nasty," Joshua said. His face had turned ashen. Jane wanted to reach out to touch him; he looked so old. "What else is in that file?" he asked.

"Copies of letters we've gotten from people, patients and staff, complaining about the cold," she said. "Including one from Mrs. LaPorte written on behalf of her husband. End of program evaluations noting the same problem. Two similar memos from the instructor and one explanatory response from administration."

"I know I'm going to be sorry I asked, but what did the one from administration say?"

"Basically, that keeping the central thermostat set at a constant level on weekends saves money and that people should be encouraged to bring sweaters."

"Shit!" Joshua exploded. "Ruth was on my case just a few weekends ago about taking my sweater in with me. What are we going to do?" The relaxed smile was now long gone. Joshua started pacing between his desk and a wall, turning sharply at the corner and returning to the desk. A triangle. Jane had seen tigers gauging the size of their cages at the zoo in exactly the same way.

Jane said, "I don't know the answer yet."

"I pay you to know the answers, damn it!"

"I know it isn't what you want to hear, Joshua, but at the moment, I don't believe anything I could say would be satisfying." Were these sudden, mercurially shifting moods of his what was frightening Mary? They certainly frightened her.

"You pay me for my considered legal judgments, not to shoot from the hip. I've got a ton of research to do tonight. I'll have a more definitive opinion for you by noon tomorrow," she said firmly. She was damn well not going to kiss his ass because *he* was upset.

"Keep me informed," he snapped. "I better get out of here before any more bad news comes along. I've had enough for one day."

He rudely pushed past her and stormed out the door not even acknowledging Mary's tentative wave good-bye.

Sixteen

The room adjoining Ruth's office was so crammed with toys it looked like a regional franchise warehouse for Santa. In the center stood a two-by-three-foot shallow box, elevated on table legs to waist height. Inside the box was four inches of smooth, fine, red sand. On all four walls surrounding the sand tray, shelves were filled to overflowing from floor to ceiling with toy-sized miniatures of everything imaginable. Baby bottles, household furniture, popular culture figures from Snow White to Darth Vader. All were gathered and displayed in categories on the walls for a person to take down and, at whim, rearrange them into a particular Lilliputian vision of the world in the sand.

Sand play, Ruth's favorite part of her practice, was a safe haven in which her clients could explore their imaginations with no restrictions imposed. All her clients who engaged in sand play had one thing in common. Somewhere in each one's childhood, the inborn joyous natural sense of play had been damaged or destroyed so that innocence and spontaneity had vanished from their adult lives. Ruth knew from personal experience how much the absence of inner freedom could undermine a human being's health.

Ruth sat in a corner of this room now and watched Lillian Roth standing, deep in thought. Her graceful hand propped up her chin while black eyes locked on the scene she'd constructed in the sand tray. Both women sat as still as sculptures in a tableau. Lillian broke the spell by placing a dog at the foot of a bridge near the middle of the scene. She paused for a moment, then turned to Ruth and said, "I'm finished with this one."

Ruth rose and came to stand next to Lillian, resting her arm on the other woman's rounded shoulder. Lillian would talk about it on her own terms. Ruth's job was to listen with all the attention she could muster.

She'd learned a lot about Lillian in the few months that they'd shared these therapeutic sessions. A pediatrician, Lillian practiced in C.C.A.'s downtown office. Lillian's husband, Ray, was a prominent lawyer in town. And although both women came from families that valued education and achievement, they'd also been sexually and physically abused by their fathers and raised in alcoholic homes.

For the better part of her therapy with Ruth, Lillian had been discovering the central imbalance in her own psyche. She now understood how her life was driven by a deep feeling of wrong-doing instilled in her by her relationship with her father, and that she had transferred this feeling to her relationship with Ray. Her sense that she was always at fault complemented Ray's needs to be in control and to criticize.

In Lillian's sand construction an adult male stood on one side of the bridge, hands on hips. He looked across at the figure of a little girl who was looking down at her feet as if in shame.

"What's happening here?" Ruth circled her hand over the man and the girl.

Lillian sighed. "Ray's been a pain in the butt."

Ruth patted Lillian's shoulder then let her arm gently drop.

Lillian bit nervously at the inside of her cheek. "He's been getting on my case. 'Too inhibited. Never loosen up.' Hell, the children and parents are at me all day long here, and then I go home to the same thing! I'm surrounded by demanding little kids from morning to night. I'm suffocating."

Ruth nodded.

Lillian curled her beetle-browed forehead. "Last night was a classic. It was his poker night with the boys. I'd just gotten into the hot tub to unwind from the day, when he comes bounding into the house. He'd decided he'd rather play with me than get drunk with the boys. Quite frankly, Ruth, I was looking forward to the time alone."

"So what happened?"

"Remember our discussion about boundaries and tough love? Well, it didn't work." Lillian paused and pulled at her brown braid.

"What did he do?"

"Put a bottle of wine and two glasses by the side of the tub, shit-eating grin on his face. Jumps in and starts playing around with me under the water. I tried to tell him as lovingly as I could that I just wasn't in the mood."

"And … ?"

"He stomped off, pouting. Fast asleep by the time I got out of the tub. Drunk was more like it." Lillian shrugged. "It feels like a no-win situation."

Ruth stole a glance at the clock and waved her hand over the middle of the box again. From among twenty examples of dogs on the shelf, Lillian had chosen a Doberman. It was frozen in a fiercely threatening stance, teeth bared, body tensed in readiness to spring. Lillian had placed it next to the figure of the frightened little girl.

"Anything more going on here you want to talk about today?"

"No, I don't think so."

The two women hugged. Lillian wasn't ready to disclose how she was planning to guard herself.

When she'd gone, Ruth grabbed the stack of pink phone messages Carla had taped to the doorjamb. Tired, she nevertheless read them. The time on the slip from Mary said six p.m. If Mary was still in the office at that hour, then Joshua's day had been no easier than hers.

"Hi, Mary. Been one of those days today, huh?" Ruth gathered her papers together, the receiver stuck under her chin.

"A day! Feels more like hell week! Make that hell month."

"Got it. Joshua's going to be late."

"I'm … uh … I'm afraid so." Mary's voice sank. "You know, Ruth, you make it so easy to talk to you—I don't have to spell everything out to you."

"Well, how long've we been doing this, Mary? I think we know the drill pretty well by now. So tell me, what's going on? I'd like to know what to expect when I go home and confront my sweetheart."

"Whatever Dr. Albert told him over lunch really set him off, for starters. He was worse when he got back from Mr. Rees' office. Now he's holed up in his office with Ms. Sherwood."

"What do you mean by set him off, Mary? I worry when you use strong language like that." Ruth couldn't help laughing to herself, even though she was beginning to get nervous. That phrase from Mary's lips was equivalent to blasphemy from someone else's.

When Ruth hung up, she was feeling a good deal shakier than she'd let Mary know. Must be one helluva malpractice suit. Joshua was usually able to contain his anger with Jane and Peter. Shouting matches behind closed doors did not bode well. She had the urge to do a sand play herself but a loud clap of thunder convinced her to start home immediately. The traffic would be awful, and she needed plenty of time to think on the way home.

Internal alarms had gone off like rockets when Mary told her Joshua had almost "ripped his office door off its hinges." It had been a long, long time since he'd displayed that kind of blind rage. But the incident was burned into her memory forever.

⚜

As soon as she'd gotten her license to practice, Joshua and Ruth tried for twelve solid months to get pregnant. By the end of the year, the humor they'd used to mask their disappointment each month began to have a stale edge to it. They agreed that she should go for a fertility test.

On the day the test results came in, Ruth walked into their living room to find Joshua in a rage, pacing the floor like a lion. He threw the letter at her feet.

"Here I am, the CEO of this fucking clinic, and those stupid assholes get your test results mixed up with someone else's! We're going back the first thing tomorrow." He towered over her. She remembered the veins in his temples, purple and pulsating. "First, I'll fire the bastard who did your test. Then I'll personally make sure they get it right this time!"

Like a movie special effect, the moment stretched and distorted everything familiar—Joshua, the objects in their living room, her briefcase still in her hand. The objects faded into nonexistence, and the sounds of the room, including Joshua's voice faded with them. Nothing was left but the hollow booming echo of her father's voice thudding in her ears.

"Lick it like a lollipop, Ruthie, and Daddy will buy you a real one."

Of course she would. She would do anything to keep her father's violent anger away. She only hoped he wouldn't force her to lie down under him. When that happened, the usual shame would be eclipsed by the searing pain between her legs.

"Don't you have anything to say?" Joshua's seemingly distant voice brought her back to herself. "Say something, for God's sake!"

"Maybe we're not getting the whole picture. Let's go in together. We can both get tested." Ruth thought fast. "It takes two to tango, after all."

That's when Joshua grabbed her cheek with one hand and raised his fist. Years of training told her that that Joshua was only acting out the script that had been written for him by his father, too. But in the heat of the moment, her own raw emotions took over. Dropping her case she lashed out and raked her nails down Joshua's cheek. She drew blood.

They stood there, looking at each other. Joshua's face had turned blanched white, the red marks where her nails had dug into him already beginning to swell and bloom a purple color. She thought she'd never seen anything so vivid.

He sunk to his knees in front of her. "Oh, my God, Ruth, I'm so sorry. I'm so sorry." He reached up to touch her cheek.

"Oh, Joshua, I am too. I am too." Tears blinded her so that his face expanded and contracted in her blurred vision. She dropped to the floor and leaned into his body, her face pressed into his chest.

"Joshua. I didn't mean to … Do you think I could ever love you less?" she whispered.

"I'll never do that again. Can you believe me?" He gently raised her face to his and kissed her.

⁓⁓⁓

Another clap of thunder wrenched her attention. Here she was, driving her car through the rain, inching her way home. She hoped to God that she could cope with anything Joshua might be bringing home tonight. If only he wouldn't shut her out again, going it alone for the thousandth time. His tendency to isolate himself when things got tough really worried her.

The answering machine was going when she finally pushed open the back door and came in out of the downpour. She dropped her umbrella and briefcase on the floor and shed her drenched coat.

"Hold on a second until I turn this infernal thing off," she panted into the phone.

"Ruth, this is Moerae. Am I interrupting something?"

"God bless you, love, how do you always know when I really need to talk to someone? You just have this thing about it. Did anyone ever suggest to you that you should go into counseling?" She sped on, unable to control her babbling. "No, you're not interrupting anything. I just walked in the door. Hell of a storm tearing up out there. And the weather isn't the only thing that's foul tonight. Mary called me before I left the office. Something has Joshua fit for bear. Mary was very upset, and you know how hard it is to get *her* riled."

"Is he home yet?"

"No. Mary said he was locked in his office having a real brawl with Jane. Evidently he'd already had two earlier in the day, one with Damien and one with Peter. He was slamming doors around. It worries me when he gets so moody."

"Has he seemed more edgy lately?"

Ruth toyed with a strand of her dripping hair. "Manic-depressive is more like it. He goes from being totally distant and preoccupied—you know, Dr. Stonewall—to wanting sex on demand. Takes one of his pills every night to sleep. It must be more than the pay-cut issue."

"Sounds like it. And when Jane canceled our afternoon of retail therapy, I figured something new was up too. But I had no idea how serious it might be until I caught the six o'clock news.

Did you catch … of course not, you just got home. Then there was Peter's phone call … "

"Never mind," Ruth cut in, hearing Joshua's car. "Unless a pilot has mistaken our driveway for O'Hare, I think Joshua has just flown in. I've got to run."

"Give me a call later if you want, dear. I'll be batching it tonight. And don't forget to watch the ten o'clock news. I'm sure they'll replay the malpractice story."

A bolt of lightning piercing the Chicago sky dramatically announced Joshua's abrupt entry through the kitchen door. He pushed past Ruth without speaking, tracking directly toward the living room bar.

"I hope that's not an omen," she said.

"Want a drink?" Joshua held up his glass in salute and downed its contents in one gulp.

"I usually wait for a man to say hello before I accept a drink from him." The way he injected that stiff Jack Daniels down his throat made her very uneasy.

"And I don't drink with women I don't know. But I gather your answer is no." He held up his glass again and raised his left eyebrow at her.

She frowned as he refilled his glass. "When Mary called to tell me you'd be late, she said you'd had a hard day."

Sensing her disapproval, Joshua went on the defense. "You might say so. In fact, it was hard enough to warrant a *couple* of drinks—at least! I believe I can make that decision for myself, thank you." He put the bottle back in the cabinet with a flourish and took a large gulp from the glass as he came back to the breakfast nook and dropped into a chair. "How was your day?"

"My day was crazy, as per usual. Thanks for asking. It's your day that sounded abnormally crazy."

"What have you heard exactly? I don't recall telling Mary anything about my business today, so it must be one of your deep throats who's coughed up. What more can I tell you that you don't know?" He cocked his head and jutted his bearded jaw at her before taking another deep pull on his bourbon.

She put her hands on her hips, walked over to the breakfast table, and stood directly in front of him, breathing deeply through her nose. "Don't even try to intimidate me. What you can talk about is what happened today that has you so upset. And don't give me any crap about how it doesn't pay to talk things out. Remember, buster: People pay to talk to me all day."

Joshua stared right back up at her, but as he stared, the creases in his brow softened. Then his whole face creased into a broad grin.

"Damn, you're a feisty bitch. I know what flared nostrils mean." One of his hands lifted the hem of her skirt an inch. His fingers felt hot on the skin of her calf. His tone softened as he teased, "But I would like to know what your fees are before I sign up, Doctor."

She slapped his hand away. "I command the highest fee there is. Rigorous and total honesty."

He caught both her hands and pulled them away from her hips drawing her close to him. "Honestly, what I need in order to handle my day is some TLC and a good night's sleep. I'm just too beat to go over it all now."

She grabbed a piece of his cheek and stared into his eyes. "Okay, peace. But let's be clear about one thing: My policy is still pay first, play later. I'll make us a tuna sandwich while you fill me in." She winked and leaned down to kiss him.

"Well, it started with a confrontation I had with Damien. Peter figured out that Damien's been in cahoots with Ashton Simons to manipulate our accounts receivables from Big Blue. How's that for openers?"

Ruth studied Joshua's smile carefully. Her patients often wore the same look of relief. Later she found they'd hoped that telling one truth would cover the need to expose another more painful one later on. She decided to ignore the warning voice telling her to pursue her hunch. "If those are you openers, I'm not sure I want to see the rest of your hand," she said, waving him to continue.

When he finished describing how Damien was selling patient data, Ruth pushed a sandwich in front of him and sat down. "Geez, he must have raked in a fortune in kickbacks on that one."

Joshua held his palm up. "We may never know exactly how much. I offered him a deal. In return for his resignation, I'll try to convince the board not to press criminal charges, but only if he'll return a chunk of money to the organization."

"That probably went over like a lead balloon." Ruth waited and watched Joshua take a big bite of his sandwich. "Joshua, what are you mulling over in your mind? I get the feeling you're holding out on me."

"You're right ... about the lead balloon. Damien didn't like it, and he intimated that he'd fight it. My guess is that means he'll try to use bad press as a threat. But what I haven't mentioned yet is that I have an ace in the hole. It looks like Damien may be an addict. The pharmacy inventory records have been tampered with." Joshua swabbed a bit of mayonnaise from his plate with his sandwich and jammed it into his mouth.

"How do you know it's him?"

"Who else could it be?" His eyes narrowed and the vein in his temple was throbbing again. Ruth wondered what was putting him on the defensive this time?

"It's a simple question. He can't be the only man in the whole outfit with access to the pharmacy's records," Ruth said calmly.

"What makes me suspicious is that when Damien installed the new computer system, he made such a big deal about a special watchdog feature he included that would protect those records

---

from unauthorized access. He's the only person who holds all the codes to get in." Joshua shoved his empty plate away, then leaned back and folded his hands across his belly.

"Hoisted by his own petard, huh? Anything else?" She picked up the plates and stuck them in the sink. Joshua massaged the back of his neck and then stroked his beard. "Oh, you mean the malpractice suit. It's the least of my worries."

Ruth felt her nostrils flaring again. "You're fidgeting with your hands, Joshua. That means you're lying to me. Are you sure the suit is insignificant?" She looked at him from the sink, her hair falling loose from the bun she'd stuffed it into for the drive home.

"Whoever your deep throat is, they're out of line calling to tell you before I've had a chance to talk to you! It pisses me off to think I can't have a private meeting in my own office without the whole world knowing what transpired before I've even finished with it!"

"When I said, 'Anything else?' I was only asking you if you wanted more to eat!" Then she added quickly, "But as for my deep throat, who has the biggest appetite for gossip among all our acquaintances? Who can you imagine was chomping at the bit to bend my ear as soon as I walked in the door the night I got home from my trip? Who never calls, but simply shows up, armed with the latest bit of dirt she can scrounge up for her own entertainment? That's right," she said, looking at Joshua sideways to see how he was accepting this diversion. "It was Elaine MacDonald."

"Given the kind of day it's been, you can imagine that a certain someone else was also chomping at the bit to get a hold on you as soon as he walked in the door. Come over here," Joshua commanded.

"Is that right? And what bit was that certain someone hoping to get hold of?" She went to him and let him put his arms around her waist.

"Well, I'll tell you what," he said, nuzzling her breasts. "Since I'm always getting heat about my need to be in control, let me practice surrender."

Ruth tilted her head. Lillian Roth's comment about taking care of children flashed briefly in her mind and she smiled. Being on top was her favorite. "Deal. I'll be up as soon as I knock off these dishes."

She stroked the top of his head and kissed his silvery hair, reminding herself to set the VCR to record the ten o'clock news before she came to bed.

⚜

Joshua took the stairs to their bedroom two at a time. Skirting the edge got his adrenalin pumping. Ruth didn't seem to take notice the few times he'd almost lost his temper. A couple of the "babies" he had stashed away in the bathroom would do the trick. He was already in bed when Ruth came up.

"Hurry up, before I change my mind," he said lazily.

"He giveth away control and then he tries to take it back. Belly up, buster. I'm driving this bus." Ruth stripped off her clothes without ceremony and crawled in beside him.

For a few minutes they simply touched. But once she was wet enough, she pushed him over on his back and mounted him, her breasts hanging and swaying gently with her rocking, brushing against his chest. Joshua's heart began pounding. He pulled her tighter onto his cock. Gripping her buttocks, he moved his head to take hold of one of her breasts with his mouth, sucking her erect nipple, rolling it with his tongue.

Ruth moaned.

"Come to me baby, come to me," he urged.

Circling her hips, she spiraled her grip on him downward, grinding her pubic hairs into his. She paused and shuddered slightly before easing her hold just enough to slide back up to the tip of his cock. She paused slightly—just enough to increase the anticipation—then plunged down on him again. Joshua had to release her nipple so he could bite his lip in an effort to stem the flood boiling in his cock. Successfully holding back, he then continued rolling her nipple in his mouth and sucking. When Ruth started panting, Joshua braced his hands under her breasts and started bucking beneath her.

"What the fuck!" he shouted squeezing her breast. He shifted her weight to the side and bolted upright into a sitting position.

"What is this?" he barked. "How long have you had this lump?" He rubbed his thumb into the area where her breast met her armpit, then reached over to turn on the bedside light.

She pulled his hand away, shook her head hard, moved the breast aside with one hand and gently rubbed the area herself.

"Let me see what you're talking about. It's probably one of those sebaceous cysts I get. You know how they tend to show up when my period goes wacky, like it has of late. It's probably just some crazy symptom of menopause."

The bourbon and halcion in Joshua's system, coupled with his guilt and shame unleashed his imagination. He stared at Ruth, but what he saw was his mother, a seventy-pound woman lying in a hospital bed in a coma. He pulled Ruth's hand rudely away and pushed her back so she was lying flat on the bed, and repeated his examination.

"What do you mean, cyst? That thing is the size of a fucking golf ball! How long have you had it?"

"For god's sake, calm down, Joshua, calm down. You're scaring me. And please, stop poking me so hard. You're hurting me too. What kind of bedside manner did you develop as an intern, anyway? I was planning to have it checked any day now, as soon as I had a free moment in my schedule. I'm sure it's nothing."

Joshua rolled over to the side of the bed and grabbed the phone. "Any day now, hell! I'm calling Peter right now!"

"Joshua, it's after ten o'clock. There's nothing Peter can do tonight. I promise I'll make an appointment to see him this week."

He stopped his furious stabbing of the telephone's buttons. He was fading fast and wouldn't be able to handle her fear on top of his own. "You're right. I'm overreacting. It just surprised and scared the piss out of me to find a lump like that. Your appointment will be tomorrow. I'll make it for you myself first thing in the morning."

Ruth rolled off the bed and grabbed her robe. "Sure, Joshua. Sure. I'm going to watch the news," she said without looking at him.

Joshua's gut tightened and his head throbbed. Is she pissed! "How about a rain check? I'll make it up to you as soon as you've had that exam."

"Sure, Joshua. Sure."

Seventeen

Joshua pulled into C.C.A.'s parking lot at four forty-five a.m. The number of cars already there surprised him. He still found it hard to believe how solid C.C.A. had become. Buzzing with activity twenty-four hours a day. He felt like a parent who wakes up one day to find his baby has grown up enough to get married.

He'd slept fitfully during the night in spite of the pills. Several times he'd awakened, shivering in a cold sweat. Once, Ruth had not been there when he jerked awake. He'd heard the TV faintly audible downstairs.

This morning he felt traumatized to the core. Everything he cared about was on the verge of blowing up in his face. Damien had to go. The only touchy part of his dismissal would be sidestepping the issue that Damien might be an addict, but Joshua was confident he wouldn't have to get into that publicly. Damien selling patient records would be sufficient cause for the board to dismiss him. And they would understand the necessity, politically, to have the whole affair handled one-on-one, just between himself and Damien. In fact, he was certain they would welcome the opportunity to avoid any confrontation.

The *Morning Tribune* bundled up at the door to the gift shop screamed their headlines. "Landmark Case Rocks Health Care!" The timing of that damned lawsuit couldn't have been worse.

The charges of managerial malpractice were ludicrous, of course. The suit was likely to be settled out of court. There was no way C.C.A. could be held accountable for Mr. LaPorte's death. But in the back of his mind there lingered the nagging memories of his own wife reminding him to take a sweater when he went to the administration building, and of his own secretary informing him about the letters complaining of the chill.

And now the lump in Ruth's breast. Ruth was probably right, nothing more than a cyst. Not the first time she'd had one. But that haunting image of his mother, shriveled into a mere husk lying in a fetal position on a hospital bed, kept flashing across his mind. So did the feeling of helplessness he felt as he watched her fade from life to death. He could never let that happen again.

Since residency, he sensed medicine involved more than just physiology and technology. AIDS patients didn't commit suicide simply because of their medical condition. People like Susan Wong needed expert bypasses *and* seeing flowers growing to heal. Breast cancer was no different. Just last week one of his colleagues had removed an ovarian growth the size of a grapefruit from a woman. Less than six months earlier, the woman's Pap tests had been clean. But three months after she'd gotten this clean bill of health, the woman's husband had suddenly left her. To Joshua's mind, a correlation existed between the woman's spiritual health and the health of her body.

He'd at least learned that much from Ruth in spite of his ritualized scoffing of her talents as a psychologist. A heart or mind that knew no peace could cause illness just as surely as a physical trauma.

The air-conditioned cafeteria sent a chill through him as he stepped in for his wake-up cup of coffee. For the moment, at least, the source of the cancer wasn't of the utmost importance. Time would make the crucial difference. He had to act at once. If the lethal cells spread to Ruth's lymph nodes, the cancer could proceed swiftly and inexorably as a runaway train, running rampant throughout her body and devouring her essence before casting her aside. No. Ruth couldn't have a malignant cancer. God wouldn't do that to him again.

During the night he'd made a desperate pact with God. If He protected Ruth and spared her life, Joshua promised to stop medicating himself. But the reality of needing to replenish his pill supply caused those panicked prayers to fade from his mind in the light of day. Joshua swallowed his coffee, scalding his tongue in the process, and left the cafeteria for the pharmacy. Still early enough. Only a skeleton crew would be on duty. If he should run into anybody, he'd plead a headache brought on by last night's news broadcast.

In a few seconds, he had restocked the cache for his empty desk drawer. He stashed an extra handful in his pocket to carry him through the next few hours until Damien's resignation could be finalized. All he needed to do now was get to his office and adjust the inventory from his own terminal. Piece of cake. He quelled the faint voice of conscience by promising himself he'd quit when all this pressure was gone.

Damien pulled into the parking lot of C.C.A. an hour earlier than his usual six a.m. check-in. But then, he wasn't supposed to be here at all. If anyone questioned him after Joshua's instructions to stay away, he'd manufactured an excuse. He'd say he only come in to check a few very important patient files. Plausible, especially after last night's news.

Damien smiled in satisfaction. He'd spent the whole night performing some very delicate work erasing every trace of anything related to Care Inc. from his office computer. The job had required great concentration, and Damien loved being thorough.

C.C.A.'s plastic surgeons weren't the only ones who could execute work so perfectly that not a shred of evidence would remain to show where the cuts had been made.

One patient record, however, required a little more tweaking before he could feel the job was completed. His own. He'd spent a couple of painstaking hours piecing it together during the night. He'd seen enough of the damn things to be able to write one up in his sleep. When his first lover, John, contracted AIDS, Damien spent days staring at his medical reports in a panic, desperately trying to find a loophole that could make the illness disappear.

He was delighted with his forgery of Scott MacDonald's signature too. That was his real stroke of genius! Like most physicians, Scott's handwriting was distinctive but nearly illegible. Damien had practiced duplicating it hundreds of times until he'd finally mastered a reasonable facsimile of Scott's scrawl—it would take an expert to see it as a forgery.

The new document he would insert this morning in C.C.A.'s patient files would be self-damning. Damien's brainstorm was to make himself out to be a victim of AIDS, having contracted the disease from John. Fortunately, it had lain dormant for so long without detection. The announcement of his resignation from C.C.A. would provide the perfect smokescreen. Joshua would be happy to say that Damien Rees was leaving for health reasons, getting C.C.A. off the hook with the media.

He needed to make a few more small but critical alterations to the two million dollar life insurance policy he'd set up when he'd originally sold his nursing home chain to C.C.A. At the time, Joshua had balked at the proposal, particularly Damien stipulating that his estate be the prime beneficiary. But Damien argued his point using Joshua's own cradle-to-grave idea of health care to drive the point home. After all, no matter how dedicated Damien would prove to be on C.C.A.'s behalf, he still needed a private life.

Now he would simply have to change the primary beneficiary on his policy to Care, Inc. Hell, no one ever got to spend his life insurance benefits anyway. Care, Inc. would perhaps issue a million dollar check to him. With any luck, he wouldn't need to give all of it back to C.C.A. and Joshua would come out looking like a hero.

As he headed toward the cafeteria, Damien patted himself on the back. It was brilliant. This whole mess could turn out to be a blessing in disguise. He quickened his pace. He'd earned a treat this morning, maybe even a sweet roll to break up his breakfast routine.

Who knows? He might even be able to tap into another hospital's records. He'd run enough scams to know how to cool out the mark—*and* to keep C.C.A. from crying wolf. No one, least of all a doctor, liked to look like a fool. Arrogant, greedy bastards. So many of them were such easy targets for any get-rich-quick scheme that came down the pike.

Care, Inc. would make a healthy profit from his insurance policy sooner or later, how much later, Damien didn't care. Everyone had to die sometime. In the meantime, if they ever tried to pressure him about the deal, he had insurance. More than enough data was stashed away in Switzerland to get them off his back. Paul was right: All Damien needed was some quiet time to figure out some loopholes.

"Hi, Mr. Rees. How are you this morning?"

"Fine, José, thank you. Give me one of those pecan rolls this morning, will you?"

José voided the register entry he'd already started to ring up. "Yogurt can get pretty tiring after a while, I'll bet."

"Yeah. I feel like something sweet this morning."

"So did the boss man. He just left here a few minutes ago and he grabbed enough sugar to feed an army."

"Must have had an emergency, I guess." Damien masked the jolt of paranoia that struck him. He came in early so that fewer people would be around to see what he was up to—especially people such as Joshua Caliban. Not like Joshua to be in at this hour.

"Don't think so." José handed Damien the executive meal slip to sign. "He seemed in no great rush to get out of here. The last thing I saw, he was ambling over toward the pharmacy, mumbling something about a really bad headache."

The comments rattled around in Damien's head as he headed for the central patient records file room. The night clerk was half-asleep. She didn't even look up as he walked by her desk.

It only took seconds to slip the new entry into his file. How many times does a man give himself AIDS on purpose? Another ironic twist in the series. He turned and walked directly to the pharmacy.

"Early in the day for a visit, isn't it, Mr. Rees?" the attendant on duty said cordially.

Waving, Damien laughed. "No. No, I'm not here to check up on you. I thought I might find Dr. Caliban here." She nodded. "Just missed him. He was by a few minutes ago. Said he had a wicked headache. Don't doubt it with the news I saw on TV last night."

"I'll bet he had a real winner. What did you give him? I may need one myself."

The attendant's casual smile disappeared. Her shoulders stiffened. "Don't know. I was busy with a rush for an ER patient, so I told him to get it himself and to leave me a note. He probably left it on the pad over by the drug destruction file. I didn't violate policy, did I? I mean, he is the president of the place and ..."

"That's okay," Damien said. "Thanks for reminding me, though. There was something specific I wanted to see in the DD's. Where did you say they were?"

The attendant pointed to a desk loaded down with papers. "Over there. Dr. Albert was in the other day looking at them, and I haven't had a chance to put them back in the drawer yet." She flushed and looked down sheepishly at her hands.

The alarms were going haywire in Damien's brain. Peter Albert. Peter Albert who'd hired that computer nerd; the same guy who'd sent Joshua after Damien's neck. What in the hell was Peter doing nosing around the DD file? Why was Joshua coming in at five in the morning to get himself something for a headache? Something in his instincts raised hope of finding that elusive ace in the hole he needed so badly. Could it be possible that he could slip the noose from around his own neck and tighten it around Joshua's?

He was so elated that he actually felt sorry for the attendant's uneasiness. "Well, as I said, I've got one specific form I have to check and then I'll be out of your way. I know you do a great job and it can be pretty thankless sometimes. What was your name?" Damien asked, peering down at the tarnished name badge.

The attendant looked up and grinned. "Wilson. Andrea Wilson. Stay as long as you'd like, Mr. Rees. Don't bother me none. Gets pretty lonely down here on the graveyard shift."

Within minutes, Damien confirmed that the last drug destruction form on file corresponded with the adjustments he'd made just the other day. That meant his records were up to date and he could investigate from home. "You're right. You guys haven't lost any stuff in several days. Good job. Thanks, Ms. Wilson."

Damien rushed to his car and winced at the sound of his starter grinding teeth with the flywheel as he hurried to get out of the parking stall. He smelled a rat in the woodpile, and the rat was a doctor to boot.

By the time he got home and turned on his computer, Damien was nearly beside himself. His fingers couldn't move fast enough on the keyboard, and the seconds required for his machine to search through and load a ton of programs seemed to crawl. The first command he gave turned on the modem in his office at work and the second gave him a printout of all the inventory changes he'd initiated in the past six months. He checked those against the drug destruction forms on file for the same time period. It was a perfect match.

He drummed his fingers on the side of his desk while he waited for the next operation to complete. The screen resolved into an intelligible format lighting up with all the brilliance of a Christmas tree.

Someone else had been making alterations in the pharmacy's inventory. All of them were made in controlled narcotics. And all had originated from Dr. Joshua Caliban's computer.

The watchdog Damien had installed in the pharmacy program had worked exceedingly well. Every time Joshua logged on to alter the inventory of one of those drugs, the troll had marked it down. How could Joshua, a computer moron, have managed to get access to an editing code that only Damien possessed? At the moment, it seemed of small consequence. Only one piece of information held any significance for him, and its importance was monumental. Joshua Caliban, the paragon of C.C.A., was a drug addict!

Damien blew his computer a kiss. An unbeatable trump card was back in his hand. He might decide that it was best to leave C.C.A. after all and set up shop somewhere else. But now that would be his decision, not Joshua's. Not only would he not have to give up the million dollars he was about to earn from Care, Inc., but he'd be able to demand a glowing letter of recommendation. His dear friend and partner would be so sorry to see Damien go.

Damien turned off his machine, stood, and stretched his arms luxuriously over his head. He'd earned his pleasure. Only an orgasm would relax the kind of energy that still charged his system like electrical fire. He'd have time to call Paul after he got done. And this phone call would be worth interrupting anything else that Paul was doing.

∻∻∻

Across town, Hal Mays had been up most of the night monitoring Damien's digital activities by remote. When Damien logged off and made his early morning excursion to C.C.A., Hal elected to grab a little shut-eye. But his mind wouldn't shut down.

Neither Hal nor Peter Albert had been surprised when Damien transferred all the suspected files to his home computer. Probably wrong technically for him to have done so, but Damien could always argue that he was only doing his job. He might even go so far as to bitch about having to take heat for being so committed to his job by taking work home. Furthermore, given the volume of patients C.C.A. cared for every day, Damien could argue he couldn't be expected to remember the specific reasons why each and every file had been brought to his attention.

Hal was pleased when Damien finally made the big mistake. Mr. Rees might be able to beat the rap about taking the records home, but his attempts to erase the entries from the watchdog program that had logged those maneuvers in the first place was a different story.

Damien would know watchdogs had been built into the system to guard against mechanical failures. He might even know about a secondary, ultra-sophisticated watchdog patrolling ethical failures, but he'd still be very hard-pressed to edit it out.

Only one or two people would ever know the codes that accessed these super-logs. In some cases, only the programmer who'd worked on the original even knew the secondary watch-dog existed. These hidden watchdogs had the very practical application of ensuring that the purchaser paid the creative developer in full for his efforts. If a contractor tried to renege on a deal, the developer could access the program and shut it down.

Damien's failure to anticipate or detect the second backup wasn't his only mistake. He'd also forgotten that he and Hal had met years before. Not that recognizing Hal would have been easy. He'd shed thirty pounds, let his prematurely gray hair grow to shoulder-length, and survived a mid-life crisis in the meantime.

But Hal hadn't forgotten Damien, or the condescending way in which he had treated his design team that helped set up C.C.A.'s computer system. When C.C.A.'s patient records were being installed, Damien had negotiated for a host of extra specs. His behavior was typical of the arrogant sons-of-bitches who thought they'd invented the damn computer only because they were so agile in manipulating it. Damien acted as if he were the only one in the universe intelligent enough to write the extra programs he wanted. He'd been a royal pain in the ass.

The rest of the project team couldn't have cared less. It meant less work for them. But Hal had instantly distrusted Damien and couldn't help loathing his pompous manner. When Hal Mays felt that way about somebody these days, he simply didn't work for him. At the time he'd met Damien, however, he didn't have that option, so he'd done the next best thing. He'd implanted a super watchdog deep in C.C.A.'s system and kept it hidden from Damien.

The universe worked in strange ways. One of the miracles it sent Hal's way was to find himself in the checkout line behind Peter Albert and his daughter, Sarah, several weeks ago. Luck, fate or poetic justice had brought Hal the opportunity to use his particular skills to terminate someone like Damien Rees. What goes around comes around.

The alarm that he'd set to wake him the instant Damien's lines became engaged suddenly went off, and he was up and fully alert.

What he discovered didn't surprise him. Damien had returned and accessed the pharmacy watchdog as soon as he turned on his modem. Both Hal and Peter had anticipated that Damien might try to cover his tracks. But oddly, Damien was making absolutely no attempt to alter so much as a single byte of the information he'd pulled up.

Why the hands-off stance with the data? Why would Damien bother looking at all, especially from the privacy of his home and in the early hours of the morning, if he didn't suspect they were on to him? Hal was sure Peter would wonder the same thing. He picked up his cellular and punched in Peter Albert's number.

Paul Blake stared at Damien's chart with some disbelief. A chart for a Mr. D. Reese should indeed be in the stack for the morning's surgery patients—but not for *D. Rees*. This was clearly a case of the files getting screwed up again. In spite of the sophistication of Damien's computer program, somewhere in the chain of events one human being would have to communicate something to another human being, and mistakes would inevitably occur.

Case in point: The medical record in his hands was for Damien Rees, not David Reese. As Damien was not his patient, Paul had no reason to review it at all. But now that it was here … curiosity overtook him—not to mention his thirst for complete control. He opened and scanned it in seconds.

Two emotions propelled the shock to his mind: A flash of sympathy for another gay brother, soon to go down. But this was short-lived, swallowed up by a blinding rage.

Thank God he and Damien had never had sex without using a condom. They had been deliberately casual about everything else in their relations, but always scrupulous about hygiene and safety. After all, they weren't serious lovers. They owed each other nothing more than a good time. Fuck the bastard. He was furious that now he'd have to make an unscheduled trip to one of those godawful sterile HIV testing centers. They were like concentration camps where people were reduced to a number.

Paul seethed with the indignity of it all. He was reasonably sure that his own health was intact. As for Damien Rees, he was going to go sooner or later. But now it was becoming increasingly clear to Paul that he preferred *sooner*. His trust in Damien was almost gone—not only did he sound like a basket case after the confrontation with Joshua, but he had actually threatened him on the phone! And to top it all off, his lover had already put him in mortal danger by withholding the fact that he had AIDS.

As Paul began to consider how he might help Damien leave both C.C.A. *and* this planet, he smiled at the fortuitous timing. After all, Damien had pretty well served his purpose in the big plan, and he had become truly expendable. But he was going to need the entire day to think through all the possible options—including a final solution.

The blinking red light told him a call was waiting on his private phone.

"Mr. Rees for you," his secretary told him.

Paul took a deep breath to calm his anger. Speak of the devil. He picked up the phone. "What's up, Damien? I'm on my way to surgery."

"Listen, I won't hold you up. At least not until tonight," Damien teased. "I've got some terrific news. I'll confirm the details today before we get together tonight. But I'm almost certain that because of what I've discovered in the last few hours, we've got Joshua by the balls."

Damien hadn't sounded this excited in months, even with all the inventions he'd introduced to their bedroom sessions. "Don't string me along, Damien. At least give me a hint."

"Dr. High-and-Mighty is a closet addict! And he gets his supply from our own pharmacy without even writing scripts. He's stealing the stuff!"

Holy Jesus! This was manna from heaven, more than he'd ever dreamed could be possible. The sky had cleared. If he played his cards right, Paul would end up with the entire pot of gold.

"Is that the greatest, or is that the greatest?"

"I'm delighted, of course. But it's almost too good to be true. Are you sure about this? Do you think you can be certain by tonight?"

"You can bet on it. I tell you, we've got Joshua on his knees. Let's have that celebration you mentioned. Be at my place by seven. Don't forget that 'something special' you were going to bring."

Paul could almost see Damien dancing in his seat on the other end of the line. "Yeah, sure. It'll be great. I've got to run. See you tonight." As he hung up, Paul smirked broadly. You can bet on it being something special.

Eighteen

Joshua watched the preparations taking place behind him from the mirror over the scrub basin. When Kathy Marshall had asked if he needed any eye drops, Joshua had been taken aback. His half-hearted joke about watching reruns of the six o'clock news all night seemed to satisfy her. So why did she keep stealing glances at him?

Holding his hands upright for Kathy to glove him, Joshua glanced over at Paul Blake. Too bad if Paul hated Joshua's constant scrutiny and avoided his eye contact. Joshua was feeling too stretched to leave anything to chance. An aortic aneurysm was the first case up, a reasonably simple ballooning of the aorta. The small and large intestines would have to be significantly relaxed, and for this purpose Paul would need to apply some healthy doses of d-tubocurarine.

Ten to fifteen milligrams injected into the I.V. would render the muscles protecting the patient's abdominal wall flaccid enough for Joshua's knife to slice easily through it. Without the relaxant, if the intestines were traumatized by an errant needle or scalpel tip, the whole mess could abruptly take on a life of its own and leap out of the patient's stomach just like a jack-in-the-box. The patient was obese and Paul had anticipated needing an extra amount.

Alongside the d-tubocurarine, Paul had his supply of neostigmine, an antidote for the d-tubocurarine. Since all of the patient's muscles would be paralyzed, the surgical team would have to keep the patient breathing by artificially manipulating his lungs. On a second's notice, the switchboard plugs of the patient's nervous system might need to be reconnected. A few milligrams of the antidote would almost instantly antagonize the curare derivative and reverse its paralyzing effects before they turned from beneficial to deadly.

Joshua nodded and the operation began. Paul pushed a few drops of d-tubocurarine out through the tip of the syringe before sending it into the IV. The patient was out, the general anesthesia already having been administered. The intermittent hissing of the respirator as it filled the air and the patient's lungs mixed with the Beethoven Joshua liked on the O.R. stereo.

The inside of Joshua's head sounded like a heated debate. Everyone was shouting at one another and at him. His attempts to control the bedlam were fruitless. The gavel he pounded reverberated through his head.

God, he was tired. So tired.

"I need some more relaxation," he said to himself, unaware that he'd actually spoken out loud.

During the momentary lulls in the chatter racing through his mind, Joshua thought he saw Paul administer another shot of d-tubocurarine to the patient. He started to say something but his attention suddenly shifted. What was Kathy Marshall doing studying the two thermo strips stuck onto the patient's forehead to monitor his body temperature and reaching under the double layer of green sheeting covering the patient's upper body to feel his arms? Was it his imagination or was the respirator having to do a little more work to keep the patient's cardiovascular system from collapsing?

248

"Kathy, what the heck are you doing feeling up the patient," he said.

"Dr. Caliban. Is it possible the patient is having a reaction to an overdose of muscle relaxant?" she asked.

"What in the hell are you talking about?" Joshua boomed.

Kathy's lower jaw dropped, forming a circle on her surgical mask. She began filling a hypodermic syringe with neostigmine. "I said, it appears as if the patient is exhibiting the symptoms of an overdose of d-tubocurarine."

Paul's hand shot out reflexively. Kathy handed the loaded hypodermic to him, then began to adjust a set of dials to deliver a booster of pure oxygen to the patient as well.

"What the hell do you think you're doing? How much have you given him?" Joshua glared at Paul.

The syringe holding the antagonizing agent into the IV was nearly empty. In a matter of seconds, the process of reconnecting the patient's downed transmission lines would be complete.

"I did exactly what you ordered, Doctor. I gave him three doses of fifteen milligrams each."

The conversations he'd been having in his head suddenly hit Joshua's consciousness with full clarity. He'd had these twilight zone experiences before. He became two people watching events unfolding but not connecting them, hearing voices but not noticing who said them, sensing but unable to make sense. But he'd never blacked out in the O.R. before. His lower jaw dropped.

Malignant hyperthermia flashed across his mind. *A very rare condition caused by combinations of general anesthetics and neuromuscular blocking agents ... almost always the result of clinical overdosage or injudicious use of curare.*

"What do you mean, I ordered? You're out of your mind!" he bellowed.

"You specifically said twice in the last few minutes, 'I need some more relaxation.'"

The tapes whirring around in Joshua's mind spun at break-neck speed. Yes, he had been complaining to himself about his fatigue. But Paul should have questioned his orders. The sight of Kathy nodding cut his automatic denial short. "Jesus Christ. If I said it at all, I was talking about myself, not the damn patient! Aren't you smart enough to tell the difference?"

"Perhaps we ought to focus on correcting the mistake that's been made instead of arguing about it," Paul said.

Joshua wasn't fooled by Paul's diplomatic unemotional restraint. Not with a face that looked as black as Paul's at that moment. His smugness was visible through his mask. Bastard. He hated Paul then, violently. His own heart was beating so rapidly he thought it might burst out of his chest. And damn it! Paul had caught him in what was absolutely the worst mistake he could make as a physician, one that had nearly cost the life of his patient. Let me humiliate myself in front of a roomful of witnesses for reasons that would have Paul Blake's best interests at heart. Scalding shame and self-loathing filled him.

Paul was his natural enemy. Why had it never been so clear until this moment? And now he'd given this vengeful predator a weapon to use against him. Not the slightest chance Paul would waste it. The only questions were when and how.

Because of his screw-up, the operation took until one-thirty before Joshua walked out of the O.R. and strode briskly to his office. Joshua's mind had refocused the instant the surgical trays were shoved aside. Now his attention jumped from one worry to another like a trained circus flea. Jane and Peter were probably already in his office waiting for him, Peter with more data from Hal Mays' surveillance and Jane with a report on her night's research. He prayed that Peter might even have the results of Ruth's lump.

Joshua leaned down to take a drink of water from the fountain outside Mary's office. As he wiped the drops that had fallen on his chin, he effortlessly slipped the pills he'd palmed from the pocket of his white coat into his mouth. Everyone would certainly have arrived. Why was his office dead silent?

Joshua burst into the office, shattering the silence.

"Rumors of the demise of C.C.A. are grossly exaggerated. Are you having a wake or a lunch? Sorry I'm late. We had a cliffhanger in the O.R. this morning," he said, making an effort at a lopsided grin.

The group offered him half-hearted smiles.

"That's okay," Jane said. "It gave us a chance to compare some notes and catch up a bit. It's been pretty hectic."

Mary stood up, averting her gaze from Joshua. She busied herself with throwing out the remnants of her lunch before heading for the door. "Thanks for letting me sit in. I'll be right outside if you need anything, Dr. Caliban."

"I'm expecting a call from Dr. Benson," Peter said to Mary. "Would you please interrupt us for it? I'm waiting for confirmation on Ruth's biopsy."

"Ditto for me, from Sam Gould," Jane called.

"What's the word, Peter?" Joshua's voice cracked slightly. "It's okay, Peter, you don't have to stand on ceremony with anyone in here." He looked around the room and noticed Moerae for the first time. "Oh, hi, Moerae. Besides, I'm always the last one to get news of importance around here. Everyone else usually gets it long before I do, so they're probably up to speed with you."

Peter said, "Ross is doing the lab work personally. We'll know exactly what her status is as soon as we hear from him, which could be at any moment."

Joshua's breath caught. "In other words, it doesn't look good and you're being a good doctor by not saying exactly that. You know I'd never sue you for malpractice, Peter."

"I'm sorry, Joshua. There's simply nothing more I can say at the moment." Peter shrugged. "I asked Moerae to organize some research for us on the relationship between organizational culture and individual behavior."

"Thank you for thinking of it," Joshua said. "Your timing, as always, is perfect. And thank you, Moerae, for responding on such short notice. We need all the help we can get. I'd rather have you on our side than testifying for the plaintiff."

"I hope you continue to feel that way, Joshua, I truly do." Moerae smiled warmly at him.

Joshua nodded, then turned to Peter. "Peter, I assume you've briefed everybody here on the situation with Damien. What's the current prognosis?"

"I called Simon Ashton to remind him that it was to his benefit as well as ours that he handle Damien in private. He huffed and puffed, but he'll deliver. I guess I'd say Ashton is in remission. Hal Mays has confirmed that Damien has been selling patient records. Damien is malignant, and unlikely to respond to radiation or chemotherapy ... " Peter stopped short as Joshua winced.

"Never mind, Peter. I can take it for now," Joshua said. He resumed control smoothly. "What's the status of our legal vulnerability, Jane?"

"Contractually, we'll have no trouble. Damien would be a fool to fight it. In the context of everything else that's going on, it's vital that we incur no additional public visibility. As we all know, the public view of the entire health care profession is at an all-time low."

Joshua smiled. "I'll take care of that one. What did you dig out last night from that ton of law books you collected?"

Jane leafed through a stack of papers. "As you might expect, the situation isn't clear-cut. The Houston case I quoted at the board retreat is the closest direct precedent I could find, and the results were ambiguous. The plaintiff's attorney got it entered in the court record that there was no performance appraisal system in place, at least not one that covered the physicians' day-to-day interpersonal behavior. However, it proved to be a moot point, because in that case the malpractice charge was medically and not managerially related." Joshua nodded.

"I called a few of my Harvard buddies last night, too," Jane continued, "and one of them told me there was a case settled out of court where a corporation was accused of murder. The wife claimed that the depression resulting from an inhumanely managed early retirement process contributed to her husband's suicide. But the most current case of any relevance involves the management of California's largest HMO and the salaries they paid themselves." Jane passed out copies of the newspaper article, and everyone fidgeted nervously as they scanned the report.

The intercom buzzed. "What is it?" Joshua asked.

"Dr. Caliban, it's Mr. Gould calling for Ms. Sherwood. And I can see Dr. Benson getting off the elevator."

"Send him in as soon as he gets here." Joshua put the speakerphone on. "Sam, this is Joshua. We're all in here together. What've you got?"

"The news isn't good. The panel voted unanimously not to require binding arbitration, just as you had suspected Jane."

"Right to the chase, Sam," Jane said. "I love that about you."

"Yeah, well, remember that in my next appraisal," Sam answered. "But seriously, I think there is a chance we can settle this baby out of court."

Jane leaned forward. "You gotta be kidding, Sam. Garth Haskins sounded like he was out for blood."

Sam laughed. "He is, but you know sharks—present company excluded—they don't care where they get it from. Garth was last seen heading off to file the motions he'd prepared in advance, and to give the press the interviews they'd requested on the way. I think he's just fanning the fire."

"We'll see," Jane said, as the knock rapped on the door. "Thanks, Sam. Hightail it back here. We've got a lot of work to do."

Ross Benson stepped in. If the man had to play poker to eat, he'd starve to death. His face gave him away before he'd taken two steps into the room. Without saying a word he walked up to Peter and handed him a manila folder with a lab report in it.

Joshua motioned for him to sit down. "You need to be apprised of what we're discussing, Ross, so if you've got a few minutes, please sit."

"It's malignant," Peter said, looking up from the report. "I'll operate the first thing tomorrow morning. I've already checked her into the hospital. She's resting comfortably."

Joshua nervously jerked out of his chair and went to the window overlooking the courtyard garden below. He pulled his handkerchief from his back pocket and wiped it across his face, then sat back down heavily.

"Moerae's research will be critical to the strength of our negotiating position," Jane finally said. "I'd like to hear from her, if that's okay with you, Joshua."

"Let me try to be as concise as I can," Moerae began. "The better someone feels about himself, the more likely he is to treat others with respect, kindness, and generosity. We know that from thousands of psychological studies. Consequently, *any* managerial policy, practice, or procedure—formal or informal—that reduces an employee's level of self-esteem contributes to potential *dis*-ease. That's because, by doing so, it's taken away the greater reservoir of tender loving care from which every patient needs to draw the strength and courage to heal.

"Documented research supports what we've known by common sense for a long time. When the providers in a health care organization suffer from poisoned relationships, it impairs how quickly and completely patients heal. Patients feel more cared for in organizations where the staff care for and respect one another, and where workers' self-esteem is enhanced rather than abused. So they heal more quickly. They require shorter hospital stays for common surgical procedures than their counterparts treated in less-caring environments."

Ross shifted in his seat. "Pardon me if this sounds ignorant, Jane. I think I'm following the direction Moerae is headed. But could you give me a practical example of how someone might use the points she's made so far in a court of law?"

Jane tapped a delicate finger on her lips. "Imagine that one of our employees injures a patient. Suppose further that that employee injures the patient because he was upset at finding out from a third party, not his supervisor, the exact reason for a recent unfavorable performance review. Or, equally as damaging, that his supervisor had delivered the bad news in a cruel and insensitive manner."

Ross held up his hand. "Wait up. Let me see if I understand you: In other words, the employee's supervisor was not being honest and direct. He wasn't telling the employee the truth to his face. He wasn't being compassionate."

"Exactly right. If the plaintiff's attorney ever got wind of our recent star-chamber fiasco, for example, we'd be easy pickings. We were not being honest and direct with one another. The argument could be made that the supervisor in question was simply following the example set by his senior executives."

Joshua asked Moerae, "Good things come in threes. Have you got anything else?"

Moerae pulled out a copy of *The Journal of the American Medical Association* from her bag. "Here's a study of the death rate of the combined 5,030 ICU patients from thirteen hospitals," she began. "The best hospital reported sixty percent fewer deaths than the documented national norm, the worst hospital reported fifty-eight percent more, and the rest fell between those two extremes. The study concluded that the differences, and I quote, 'appear to be related to the quality of the interaction and communication between physicians and nurses'."

Moerae looked around the room. Joshua looked confident, smiling engagingly at her as if she were a prize prodigy who'd performed well for her tutor. Everyone else looked as though they'd just been punched in the stomach.

Peter asked, "By that set of standards, there isn't a health care organization in existence that's immune to charges of managerial malpractice, is there?"

"Jane is in a better position to speculate on how the courts might view the picture I've tried to paint," Moerae said.

"This is purely speculative," Jane said, "but I'd say the primary point of vulnerability lies in the absence of any systematic attempt on an organization's part to hold people accountable for the consequences of the healing quality of their day-to-day behavior."

Joshua felt himself crumple under the gentle weight of Jane's words. His shoulders sagged and his hands trembled. Moerae's amber eyes radiated sympathy. When he started to speak, his mouth was so dry the words came out in a ragged rhythm. Why were they sticking to his tongue? "We can't do any more than we do now with practice review committees, can we, Ross?" he asked.

"We can't afford to chase windmills, my friend," Ross said shaking his sleekly combed silver-grey head. "I don't think Moerae and Jane are talking about the technical effectiveness of the medicine we practice. There's no question that it impacts the curing of disease in a positive way. I think what they're talking about is the effect of our personal behavior as doctors and administrators. I fear we really hurt clinical outcomes with our sometimes selfish and self-centered conduct."

Joshua's breathing labored. In the air-conditioned chill, his skin prickled with sweat, the tightness in his neck not responding to his vigorous rubbing. "Maybe my father was right. I'd have probably been better off going into the car dealership business instead of a care dealership."

Moerae looked at him carefully. "Would it be of any help to know that it's only a matter of when, not if, the issue catches up with car dealerships?"

Jane, Ross and Peter leaned toward her.

"Sure, go ahead. Misery loves company," Joshua said.

"Actually, Joshua, I think this might give us some useful bargaining chips at some point, though I'm not even sure how. Managerial behavior in today's world reflects the following belief: Treating employees well—and often customers—stands in direct conflict with the bottom line. Most businesses believe that the more money spent on employee development, the smaller the profit will be.

"There's no other way to explain the regularity with which organizations slash their human resource development budgets in the face of declining economic returns. If people truly were seen to be the most important asset of an organization, management would increase the investment in their employees, particularly when the going got tough. But organizations don't act that way at all."

Joshua shifted uneasily. Didn't Damien just report that he'd butchered the staff training and development budget to the bone, but hadn't touched the doctor's kitty?

"If organizations truly believed that dollar profits and investments in human resource development are in conflict," Moerae went on, "then they would have to admit that a certain amount of self-esteem has to be sacrificed whenever a commodity or service is produced, because a dollar's profit comes at the expense of a piece of the human spirit. What would happen if truth in advertising required product labels to state clearly how much self-esteem went into its making as well as how much salt, fat, and cholesterol?

"Companies ought to be required to disclose to prospective employees the same facts. 'Here are your job requirements: Duties, time and a certain amount of your spirit.' Salary and benefits can only compensate a worker for the investment of his mind and body. It can neither purchase nor repay investments of heart and soul. It can't buy love."

"The next thing you know, somebody will be bringing a malpractice suit against the oldest profession in the world," Joshua said. Everyone laughed, draining the tension from their tired faces. "Let's knock it off for now. Ross, I'm glad you could sit in on this. Do the best job you can of containing the rumor mill in this place.

"Moerae, what you've told us backs us into an uncomfortable corner! But I'm grateful—*really*—grateful, to have you in that corner with us.

"And Jane, you'll have to work out something for me to say to the press by the end of the day tomorrow." He looked at each of them to see if there were any questions. Each one nodded. Joshua sighed. Was that really fondness for him he saw in their eyes?

"Good. Then I'm going to visit a very special patient we've just admitted."

"I'll walk up with you," Peter said.

"I should hope so. You're her doctor." Joshua draped his arm affectionately over Peter's shoulder.

Nineteen

With his back to Mary's desk, Peter Albert stood at the window outside Joshua's office watching the clouds change shape with mercurial speed outside. His emotions had gone ballistic when Hal telephoned a second time this morning to tell him that inventory records in controlled narcotics had been adjusted just fifteen minutes earlier. And, the editing had come from Joshua's desk, not Damien's. The man he most loved and trusted had betrayed him. Would the churning in his stomach ever quell?

Jane and Moerae had gone, leaving Joshua to excuse himself while he disappeared into his private bathroom for a few minutes before joining Peter. This diversion only served to deepen the pain that gripped Peter's heart. Joshua had looked like a man scrambling up the face of a glass cliff. Peter was sure Joshua would be fortifying himself with some of his chemical helpers right now.

Confronting Joshua was going to be hell. But—with God's help—managing all the other problems jeopardizing C.C.A.'s well-being depended on resolving this one. And Ruth. How could he take a knife to Ruth tomorrow if this thing with Joshua wasn't resolved today?

He jumped when he heard Joshua's voice behind him.

"Are you all right, Mary?"

Peter turned to see Joshua leaning over his secretary's desk, his hand on Mary's shoulder. For the first time, Peter noticed her reddened eyes and the wet patches on her cheeks and chin.

Mary dabbed her eyes with a handkerchief. She seemed unable to speak.

"Mary, ignore what I've told you in the past about my not wanting to play poker with you. You couldn't bluff if your life depended on it," Joshua chided her. "What's up?"

"I'm sorry, Dr. Caliban. Mrs. Caliban dropped by this morning. Before going to see you, Dr. Albert. And I'm just … I'm just frightened, for both of you. When I saw the look on Dr. Benson's face, I knew it wasn't good news."

"No, the results weren't good," Peter said quickly. "But Mary, you know how important it is that Ruth has the support and love of people like you. It will help bolster her courage if we can all be as honest as we can with her. If you get a chance, please stop by to see her before you go home."

Joshua frowned and tilted his head, as if he weren't sure he wanted to hear the whole truth yet. "She'll be fine, Mary," he said, but his assurance had a hollow ring to it. "After all, she has the best surgeon in the business. Do you have anything for me before I go over to see what kind of job he's been doing so far?"

"This came in the morning mail," she said, handing him a letter.

Joshua fingered the hand-addressed envelope. Printed boldly on the front were the words PERSONAL AND CONFIDENTIAL from Mr. and Mrs. Henry Wong. He stuffed it into his shirt pocket.

"Thanks, Mary. Page me if you need me, but only if it's a real emergency."

Peter could hardly believe his ears. What else could possibly happen to warrant Joshua calling it a *real* emergency? Suddenly he noticed a book lying on Mary's desk. Me of little faith. Thank you, God.

"How do you like this book, Mary?" he asked.

"Very much, Dr. Albert," she said. Her chocolate eyes peered at him over her bifocals. "It's a very inspiring story."

"I just finished reading it, myself. My wife told me about it. And I agree, it's very inspiring." It was about Sacajawea, Lewis & Clark's guide, a proud Shoshoni woman of high rank and deeply revered by her people. Peter was thinking of a specific account in the book that told of a time Sacajawea was deathly ill. As she lay lifelessly by a fire gone cold, the most powerful medicine man in the village was called in to heal her.

He felt her head and placed his ear to her breast. Then the medicine man walked twenty paces from her and called for his bull whip. The crowd that had gathered to watch him gasped in shock as he snapped the knotted tip of the leather strap in the air a mere hair's breadth above Sacajawea's eyes and sunken cheeks.

The medicine man did this again and again until the princess's body stirred on the ground. Her cheeks grew pink, but the crowd couldn't see if the whip had actually touched her and drawn blood to the surface.

Three more sharp snaps of the whip and suddenly Sacajawea's hand struck out with the swiftness of a snake to grab the end of the whip. The medicine man fell to his knees and chanted a prayer of thanks that the will to live had returned to warm the frozen heart of their beloved Sacajawea.

Would he be able to renew the will to live in Joshua by cracking a figurative whip in his face? He could risk the wrath he was sure to incur by confronting Joshua with his addiction, because only the pure raw energy of rage had the power to burn through Joshua's defenses. That done, he could guide his friend through

---

his anger to surrender and acceptance. Then healing was possible.

"Let's take the outside route to the hospital," Peter said as he and Joshua started off to see Ruth. "I could use a breath of fresh air."

"Me too. I feel like I'm on the backlash of a fishing reel."

"For me, the metaphor is a hornet's nest. I don't know how you cope. What do you do to keep from going crazy?" Peter tried to calm his nerves, but he couldn't look at Joshua.

"The malpractice suit will sort itself out," Joshua started off. "I have complete confidence in Jane, and Moerae will be of great help. She's proven that today. It's the situation with Damien that has me the most concerned."

Peter locked his hands behind his back. This wasn't going to be easy. Here they were, on their way to see Ruth who had a malignant cancer, and Joshua's concern of the moment was Damien. "What are you planning to do about that mess?"

"The Big Blue piece is in hand. I told Damien I might be able to prevail upon the board not to press charges on the insurance scam if, in return, Damien gives us some financial restitution. The board will be happy with the windfall. I figure what's done is done. The families got what they voluntarily signed up for. Maybe we can salvage something of lasting value for future patients. If Damien squawks, however, I've got him cold with the drug stuff."

"Let's have a seat for a minute." Before Joshua could protest, Peter grabbed his elbow and pulled him firmly toward a secluded bench under a shade tree in the courtyard. "Ruth will still be a little groggy from the anesthesia. We can take a few moments."

"Okay, but just for a minute. I'm anxious to see Ruth."

"Tell me, how did Damien take it when you questioned him about the narcotics inventories?"

"Well, I decided the best strategy was not to let on to Damien that we had an ace up our sleeves. I'd rather wait until we're forced to show our hand. Have you uncovered anything new?"

"I've got a lot of unanswered questions, and that's about it."

"I've got a few myself. What did you hear from your computer wizard?" Joshua asked.

"Well, Hal confirmed that the narcotics inventory had been tampered with as recently as early this morning."

"Of course it was," Joshua shot back. "How else would Damien be able to cover his tracks? And I thought I told that bastard to stay home for a few days."

"That's something else I've learned. All of these changes can be made from any computer with a modem as long as you know the access codes."

"No system is too hard for Damien to break into, is it?" Joshua said. "Particularly one he helped to design."

Peter realized it was pure fantasy to think Joshua was going to open up on his own. He looked directly at him and took the plunge.

"What has me thoroughly confused is why Damien, or whoever else has the access code, would be so careless as to access the log only from your computer?"

Joshua stood up abruptly. He gritted his teeth, his jaw bulging. A vein in his temple pulsed visibly but he tried to keep his voice down.

"If it wasn't for the fact that I need you to operate on my wife tomorrow, I'd break your fucking neck for what you're implying. I've told you before you had big balls for a little guy, but don't let your bravery go to your head. Until I tell you otherwise, I'm still the boss around here."

The boil has been lanced and now Peter could begin. He felt amazingly light, as if a pound of lead that had been coursing through his veins was emptied out all at once.

"This isn't about locker room pecker-checking, Joshua. And, just for the record, I'm not interested in your job. In fact, I'm ready to resign from mine effective this minute if necessary." Peter sat up straight, shoulders relaxed. He continued to gaze unwaveringly into Joshua's eyes. "This is about two people whom I love and respect. One of them will be on my operating table tomorrow with a cancer in her breast. The other is you, the head of C.C.A. I love this organization as much as you do, but it'll need a heart transplant to survive and it's you who'll have to be the surgeon. I'm talking about how both our minds are going to be clear and how our hands are going to be steady when we approach our respective operating rooms. You can trust me on this. I'm not taking the knife to anyone, least of all Ruth, until this issue is straightened out between you and me. You're going to have to come out of hiding, Joshua."

Joshua leaned forward for a second, grabbing the branch of the tree overhead before he slumped back onto the bench. He rubbed his face hard with one hand, over and over again, from his forehead down to his jaw.

"You're serious aren't you? I mean, about quitting right now, before you operate on Ruth."

"It's not meant as a threat, Joshua. I'm saying I can't trust myself as long as I feel so unsettled about you. Ruth deserves the best I can give, but I can't deliver until I know what you plan to do."

Joshua wiped a tear from his cheek. When he spoke, his voice was barely audible. "Everything is falling apart at the seams, Peter. The stress … got to me, and I let it get a little out of hand. Can't we talk about this after we get our heads above water? Why do we have to address this now, Peter? Why now? Can't we hold off for a while?"

"I can't do that without undermining my self-respect, Joshua, and I need that to keep the knife steady in my hand. I love you and Ruth too much to ignore what's going on with you any longer. I've already let it go too long. I didn't want to admit what was going on with you even to myself. Now I can't believe it's beneficial to prolong the agony, and that's what we'd be doing if we postpone facing up to these things. The truth will set us free, Joshua. Even though it's going to put us through an unimaginable emotional wringer, it *will* set us free."

Joshua's eyes were focused on the space between his shoes, his head hanging. He sighed, swallowed a deep breath, and looked at Peter. "Are you willing to see me through it? What do you want me to do?"

Peter took both of Joshua's hands in his and suddenly Joshua felt a little lighter, a little freer.

"If you'll take some time off by yourself to think it through, I can trust you to do what's right. I want Ruth to rest as much as possible tonight. Why don't you go up to the cabin? It's only an hour and a half away. You can fish some, get a good night's sleep, and still be back here by seven in the morning. I won't start surgery until about seven-thirty. You can buy me breakfast," he smiled, "since I'm not billing you for my services."

Joshua got up from the bench, still hanging on to Peter's hands. "But that doesn't mean it's for free. It took guts for you to speak to me with an open heart. Whatever it cost you in courage to face me, I know I'll have to measure up in kind."

"Unless I miss my guess," Peter said, glancing up behind him at the wing where Ruth's room was, "your wife is waiting for you." He squeezed Joshua's hands and let them go.

Framed in a window three floors up, Ruth waved her hands, beckoning.

"Let's go up," Peter said. "I don't want my patient satisfaction ratings to fall anymore by making you late."

⁓⌇⁓

From her vantage point, Ruth could only guess what the two men were talking about, but as she watched, she actually wondered if they might come to blows. Even from her distance she could see the tension knotting up in her husband's body, bunching under his shoulders like an animal ready to pounce. And Peter was so stalwart, seeming to move in closest just at the moment of greatest danger. Could she be as strong when she confronted Joshua herself?

She hadn't slept a wink last night. She lay on the couch all night, pissed at Joshua for drugging himself to sleep, and berating herself for her stupidity. Married to a doctor, working in a clinic, and she couldn't find the time for regular checkups. Too busy to pay attention to the tenderness she'd felt in her breast.

As a psychologist, Ruth understood her breasts represented: generosity, protection and comfort, all things that are associated with mothering. Physiologically, the possible causes weren't entirely within her control, but the possible emotional sources of her disease, which stemmed from attitudes and behavior, *were* within her power to control. Her relationship with Joshua, for example, was undermined with the poison of lies and deceit that both of them had committed. Joshua had hidden his dependency on drugs from her. She had hidden her anger at his pattern of withdrawal. Easier to preach tough love to Lillian Roth than live it herself.

It wasn't only she who'd paid dearly either. Joshua's price was steep. The feminine side of his nature was underdeveloped, stuck. He'd turned to drugs, alcohol and the destructive macho game of competition as his sources of self-nurturing. He'd developed an unhealthy fantasy about C.C.A., substituting it for the son he'd never fathered. It was very possible that he would lose it, his greatest hope and joy, for failing to balance the elements in his soul. And if she couldn't help him to see this in the next hour or so, he might have to forfeit his marriage as well.

Joshua's voice echoed in the hallway. She slid onto the hospital bed and pulled the sheets over her legs. He would be anxious when he opened the door. She wanted to be composed from the first moment he saw her, but damn it, the tears wouldn't stop streaming down her face.

He was such a large man that his entrance into a room was always an event of significance, but oh how he sagged when he opened the door. The lines under his eyes were couched in dark folds and his wide, generous mouth was pinched into a seam. A tic twitched in his cheek.

At first, he appeared not to really see her. When he did, he stopped and reached out to lean on Peter. What could be going through his mind? Was he seeing his mother, propped up in the bed, ghostly and glowing in the white glare of the sheets? Or was he really seeing her, alive, but throbbing with the pain of all their mistakes?

Peter let Joshua lean against him for a second and then pushed past to come to Ruth. He placed one hand tenderly on her forehead and grabbed her wrist with the other. He nodded to Joshua. "Vitals fine."

Joshua moved away from the door and came to the other side of Ruth's bed. He leaned down to kiss her lips. He stroked the tears from her face with his thumbs until she reached up and pulled his face back for another kiss.

"I love you, sweetheart," she said. "Give me a minute to talk to my doctor so he can earn his keep. Then we'll throw him out of here. He doesn't really need me until tomorrow."

"How did you know the operation was scheduled for tomorrow morning?" Peter asked. "Has somebody violated the doctor-patient relationship, or did you pull rank and drag it out of some hapless nurse before I could get here to tell you?"

"Neither. Just call it woman's intuition. Plus, I do know something about a surgeon's schedule."

"Ruth, it's very important that you fully accept the whole situation now," Peter said solemnly. "As far as I can tell, this cancer hasn't been growing for very long, but it has been growing rapidly. That's why I think we should proceed with surgery immediately."

"So, are you telling me I should say good-bye to my breast tonight?" she asked.

"At least a piece of it. Until I take a closer look, I won't know how much. But you know what they say … "

"Yeah, as long as it's big enough to get your hands around, or put into your mouth, it's good enough. And that saying's good for us women, too," Ruth finished for him.

Peter clapped his hands and laughed heartily. "God, I knew it! Women talk about the same things in the locker room as we do. I'll be back tonight before I go home. We can talk about the details of the surgery then, if you want."

"That'll be fine," she said, managing a smile. "I'd like some time with Joshua alone, now, if we can make an exception about visiting hours."

Peter planted an affectionate kiss on her forehead. "I'm sure the president of this place won't mind. I must warn you, however, that as your doctor, I've prescribed that he make himself scarce tonight. I'll see you later."

Joshua stood by Ruth's side, frowning and kneading her hand between his. He sighed heavily, tears in his eyes.

"I need to take a piss," he said huskily. "I'll be right out."

The toilet flushed. It took a full two minutes for him to turn off the water from the tap, longer than to simply wash his hands. Throwing water on his face, no doubt. Ruth gritted her teeth. She knew when he emerged, his face would bear no traces of weakness. He'd be in control again. But for her, the mask was painfully transparent.

"It sounds like Peter's pretty optimistic about the situation."

Ruth took a deep breath. He was standing over her, holding her hands again. She released them and pushed his hands gently but firmly from her.

"Which situation are you referring to, Joshua? Damien? The news broadcast? Or my breast cancer? And how dare you refer to my breast as 'the situation'?"

Joshua tightened his fists and bit his lip. "You know what I meant, Ruth. You have a right to be frightened and angry. But everything will be fine, you'll see."

"Yes, I'm very frightened, Joshua. I'm not looking forward to having a part of my breast removed. Or the treatments I'll need afterwards. But frankly, what scares the crap out of me is that you haven't been honest with me."

Joshua swayed. "There's so much going on … I'm having trouble keeping track of everything all at once, myself. Feeling that lump on your breast last night shook me up, too, you know."

"Do you remember what I told you last night, that I command the highest of fees? That I demand rigorous honesty? Well, in the last twelve hours I've had to be honest with myself about a lot of shit. Some of it is my responsibility to clean up," Ruth said.

"Like what, for example?"

Ruth's nostrils flared. Trust him to deflect the spotlight away from himself. "I'll give you one example, but then we'll focus on your shit. Because if you want to see me after my operation tomorrow, you're going to have to come clean." He reached out to touch her face, but she warded off his hand. "And I don't want any sympathy from you, buster, for my tears right now!"

"Boy, you really are pissed about something." His face was slowly crumpling.

"You've got that right. I'm furious with myself, first of all, for never having the courage to talk with you about even the possibility of adopting a baby."

———

Joshua's jaw dropped. "I never even suspected you thought about it!"

"My point exactly, Joshua. I'm not saying I want one now. I doubt that I do. What I am saying is that I won't participate any longer in a relationship where those kinds of things go un-discussed. I will not agree to there being so little real communication between us anymore. You didn't tell me the whole truth about what was going on last night. You held out on me in a major way."

Joshua's hand reached up to loosen the collar on his already opened shirt.

"Getting nervous? As well you might," Ruth growled.

"In the face of what was happening to you, it didn't seem relevant to bother telling you about Damien's drug problem."

"Joshua, I looked in your office desk drawer this morning," Ruth said evenly.

For a moment, Joshua didn't move. Then he smashed his fist explosively down on the bed. "You have no right to be nosing around in my desk drawer!"

"That's true. And two wrongs don't make a right," she continued. She was beyond intimidation. "But the critical point is, you have no right to lie that way to me or to yourself. Your pills have become your mistress, damn it! You confide in them more than you do in me. You seek their comfort, not mine, when you feel the need for support. So every time you tell me you love me, those words come out through a smokescreen of deception. I realize now that every time I swallowed one of your lies, I helped to feed the cancer in my breast. I won't have that kind of poison in our relationship any more. Do you understand me? *It's over*. I won't have it in my recovery room, either."

Joshua jumped out of his chair as though he'd been stuck with a pin. He lurched unsteadily over to the window. For several minutes he gazed silently out onto the courtyard below, trembling from head to foot. Ruth could see him gathering his forces, and wasn't surprised when he spun around and roared at her in helpless rage. "You hung my dirty linen out for Mary and the whole world to see! With everything else that's going on, you've ruined me. How am I going to save this place when everyone is running around telling on everyone else? I just let my stress get a little bit out of hand, that's all."

"Don't you see, my love, you're still lying to yourself?" she said. The tension had gone from her. He would probably choose to go through the struggle alone. "You've told me yourself, Joshua, that we're not gods. The best we can do is try to save ourselves. There are many, many people who love you. You don't have to go through this alone."

"I've been alone all of my life, Ruth," he said slowly. Tears were beginning to wash down his face. "And now you're threatening to abandon me when I need you most."

Ruth held out her arms to him. Joshua hesitated, then staggered to her side. She waited for him to sit beside her and drew his head up against her breast.

"Joshua, I love you. The last thing I want to do is abandon you. Whatever gave you that crazy idea?"

"You told me you didn't want me to be there in the recovery room tomorrow."

"I *do* want you there. I *need* you there. I don't want to open my eyes after losing a part of my body and not see your face. But what I need is you, the man I love, not some stranger whose identity depends on chemicals to keep him standing up."

"I'm sorry, sweetheart. I'm sorry."

She'd been around the block enough in her professional life to see he wasn't at his bottom yet. She prayed it wasn't too much further down. But this was a start—a good, solid start.

"I'm sorry too, sweetheart. It hasn't been all your fault. I've more than played my part by letting you go on without challenging you. It does take two to tango."

"That's not what you just told your doctor."

"Huh?"

"All you need is something you can get your hands around or into your mouth," he said.

She laughed with delight. "Let's say good-bye to it properly, then. She deserves at least that much."

Joshua opened her nightgown and put his mouth over the cancerous breast as Ruth stroked his head. For the moment, she felt secure.

Twenty

Paul settled into his high-backed, suede-covered swivel chair. How superbly everything was going for him! Thank God he'd demanded that his portion of the insurance kickbacks be paid in cash, for now there would be no checks that could be traced back to him. He felt invincible—like one of those medieval knights heading off to the Holy Land wearing forty pounds of steel armor. Damien, like Joshua, would be sorry he'd ever threatened Paul.

He scuffed his stockinged feet through the thick white carpet on the floor and sighed with pleasure. The carpeting and the soft gold brocade paper covering the walls were not only beautiful, they also softened the acoustics in this room he'd converted into his private recording studio.

He removed a tape from the editing machine. The thousands of dollars invested in this equipment would be worth more than he'd put in. Paul could piece together virtually any conversation he wanted, as long as his raw data was good.

"Ummm. Oh, I like that a lot."

Elaine MacDonald's voice was as husky and warm as a fuzzy summer peach. Paul closed his eyes so he could replay the whole scene.

"Oh, yeah? What do you like about it?"

"I love feeling your cock rubbing up against my panties. I love seeing the little spot of wetness you make. "

"What else do you really like? "

"Hmmm. When you pull the backside of my panties together so that they're hidden in the crack. That really turns me on."

"Your wish is my command. And then what would you do next?"

"And then I would rip my panties off of your body and eat whatever I found wrapped inside. "

"Keep going, I—I'm coming. "

Paul stopped the tape, rewound it a short bit, and replayed a part of it. Very satisfying. A simple little cut and tuck, splicing a phrase borrowed from one part of the taped conversation to another, and he had a seamless little vignette from an afternoon dalliance to add to his collection.

Paul got the idea for this little 900 number business years ago, when he and his college buddies used to tape other people engaged in various erotic pursuits and bodily functions as a fraternity prank. A tape recorder planted in the bathroom garnered them unlimited raw footage of men and women caught in their most private moments. The tapes were great for laughs, or even a little gentle persuasion when someone was reluctant to put out. But the most valuable lesson learned was that most people would pay to protect their privacy.

Paul had a taste for blackmail. He expanded his repertoire and went commercial with it when he sold a tape he'd made of the dean of the school getting it on with her husband's best friend in the frat house spare bedroom. After that, it was a simple progression to his "900 number show" which provided callers with any kind of auditory turn-on they wanted, erotic or scatological. The name he'd chosen, From Real To Reel, tickled his fancy—it was clever and a little "retro." It reminded him of the good old days and their massive reel-to-reel tape recorders.

The red light of his private line began to flash silently on the wall beside him.

"Hello. Dr. Blake's residence."

"Is this the Dr. Blake of fame, fortune, and infinite staying power?" Elaine crooned in his ear.

Paul stifled his irritation. He'd asked her a dozen times to be more discreet on the phone. But he'd need an alibi for tonight's games with Damien, and Elaine would fit the bill. He had to soften his answer.

"That depends on where you'll be staying for a few hours tonight."

"You're in luck, and everything that rhymes with it! The doggie is out of town. He's not due back in until late tonight."

"I'll be over in thirty minutes."

"Not so fast. When you're hot, you're hot, Elaine, that's what I like about you. But sometimes you just go over the edge—too pushy, do you know what I mean? So listen up. I've got an earlier appointment, but I should be back here by eight-thirty at the latest."

"Darling, I hate to whine, but that doesn't give us much time. Scott'll be home by midnight. Besides, you know how I hate being sloppy seconds. You know how much I love to fuck you. Is there someone else?"

"Don't be coy, Elaine. It's not becoming. You know I thrive on diversity, but no, there isn't anyone else tonight," he lied.

"It's a business meeting. Even if it wasn't, I always save the best for you. Just like you do for me."

"Okay, but I don't want to be hanging around by the phone waiting for you to get home. Leave me a number where I can reach you in case Scottie should change his plans at the last minute."

"You're pushing it, Elaine." He hated this aggressiveness in her, but, like him, she loved skating just on the edge of their being discovered. The tension added spice to the sex. And he wanted to stay in her good graces tonight. "All right, I'll give you a private number where I can be reached. If you call and I'm not there, at least use a code signal."

"Okay. If for some reason I can't make it, if Scottie decides to come home early, I'll just say the cupboard's no longer bare."

"That's fine. Just don't get impatient. I'll call you on my car phone as soon as I leave my appointment. And I'll have a little surprise for you." That last tidbit would drive her crazy with anticipation.

"Oh, God. Do you mean it? Is it the same stuff you had before?"

"That's for me to know and for you to find out. I'll see you later. "

He packed his black bag. One recorder, carefully checked and stowed. A healthy supply of other goodies: yohimbine, cocaine, a few treats for himself, several clean needles, and the special surprise he'd promised. On second thought, he put in some extra yohimbine.

Elaine was hot so he'd need enough for both sessions tonight. It was one of those drugs that wasn't available to just anyone, for it required a skillful practitioner to inject it into the femoral artery, just above the groin. The blood carried it to the pelvis, causing a man's penis to pop up like a jack-in-the-box, rock-hard. And it would stay that way as long as thirty minutes. Yohimbine had always guaranteed the greatest pleasure to himself and his partner, male or female. Thinking of this, Paul put a second recorder in his pants pocket.

The mirror in front of his closet reflected his laughing image as he stood there running his fingers over the soft cool sleeves of the fancy shirts hanging the full length of the upper closet. He had something to wear for every occasion, from a surgical procedure to a wake.

But he'd never dressed for a murder before.

❦

Damien had been working feverishly all afternoon to get ready for the evening's celebration. Yohimbine was truly a miracle drug. The first time Paul brought it, Damien thought he would die. Paul coaxed him plenty, and pumped him with enough coke to erase his fears, however, so he allowed Paul to put the needle in his stomach. After that, he never looked back.

Damien had gone all out for this occasion, splurging on several new toys in a deliciously indulgent shopping spree that afternoon. He laid out a new set of handcuffs and the vibrator he'd bought on the massage table in his bedroom, and admired their reflections in the sparkling new mirror he'd installed on the ceiling. The piecè de resistance was the exquisite set of silk sheets. Their slithering, coolness on his naked body would drive Paul totally crazy.

The chief reason for this burst of extravagance was that the morning had progressed as if on oiled wheels. The meeting with Care, Inc. had been tense, but once Damien made it clear what kind of information he'd tucked away, their board had capitulated. The million bucks threw them for a loop. Damien had been brilliant, working himself up to tears for his lost love John, and when he explained he had no family to inherit his estate, Care, Inc.'s own greed settled the matter. The idea of making a cool million dollar profit in a matter of months was very seductive.

Added to this triumph, Damien made the unbelievable discovery that, while he was out, Joshua had made several withdrawals from the narcotics inventories. Dr. Caliban would soon be out of his hair.

Damien smoothed the new sheets and then jumped onto the bed like a little kid on a trampoline. He lay with his hands behind his head, staring up at the mirrored image on the ceiling. He resembled a kind of elegant, black-clad starfish pinned to the round waterbed. A pile of plump pillows spilled over the edges of the bed and seemed to melt in a sea of thick, red-and-white carpet.

A little touch of the grotesque put everything else into perspective, and to achieve this end Damien had blown up several condoms and hung them like balloons around the bedroom. He reached up and ran his fingers over the surface of the black, flocked wallpaper that had always made him think of closely cropped pubic hair. Once, Paul had commented that all the room needed to look like a huge asshole from a helicopter was pink sheets on the bed. He was right.

Paul. Ever since John's death, Damien had never allowed himself to fall in love. Sex for convenience, sex for pleasure, sex for fun, but never sex for seriousness. Paul and Damien had been very clear from the beginning that the only way their relationship would work was to make no commitments. So far, they'd been successful. But recently Damien had entertained fantasies of disappearing with Paul and the million bucks from Care, Inc.

Damien loathed confusion. Were these fantasies driven by loneliness? Fear? Or was he actually falling in love again? How much could he really trust Paul? Paul had withheld events from the closed board meetings and that niggled at him. But then, wasn't he lying to Paul about his AIDS? He was cool. He would play it by ear and see how Paul would react to Joshua's imminent demise.

The security buzzer hummed at seven p.m. sharp. Paul was always a stickler for being on time.

"Mr. Rees, Dr. Blake is here to see you," Tony, the building concierge, announced.

"Send him right up, Tony. And, Tony, we've got some important work to do, so will you please see we're not interrupted this evening?"

"Got it. No outside interruptus this evening."

Damien smirked. "I count on your discretion."

Damien remembered one more detail. Yes, the three new porn videos were there by the console. An orgy for any persuasion gay, lesbian, or bi. Damien thought Paul was nuts to want sex tapes playing when he was having the real thing, but he couldn't deny they turned Paul on—spectacularly.

He'd learned a lot of new tricks from Paul, come to think of it. Paul loved to talk dirty and was so good at it, it had become contagious. Now even Damien was experimenting with rude talk during their private sessions together. Yes, Paul had brought something special into his life again. Maybe he'd risk trying for love again.

The sensation of the elevator shooting up the shaft to Damien's penthouse paralleled the adrenaline pumping through Paul's body. He reviewed his plan again. If he worked quickly, he could get rid of Damien in time to meet Elaine no later than eight-thirty. That shouldn't be a problem. He was adept at giving shots, and it'd be even easier to give Damien his surprise because he'd be eager to take it.

The hard part would be steering the conversation in the right direction for Paul to reconstruct it later into a plausible suicide tape. Damien was already sounding giddy on the phone earlier and Paul knew how to loosen his tongue even more.

Once he got Damien going, he'd trigger the recorder in his pocket, sit back, and relax. Paul pressed the button at Damien's door and took a deep breath. Damien's footsteps paused on the other side of the door, probably touching up the flower arrangement he kept in the hallway.

"Hang on, Paul. I'm coming."

Paul came in and waited until Damien closed and chained the door before he took Damien in his arms and kissed him. Damien reached behind Paul and squeezed his ass. Paul broke away first. He always did, but this time he had a schedule that made him extra antsy.

"Let's get business out of the way before we get too wrapped up." He looked with amusement at Damien who was almost dancing on his feet with anticipation. "Come on, man, get a grip on yourself. You're acting like a kid in heat, and a green one at that. Like somebody who's never been laid before."

"All right, all right. Business first. But let's smoke a little grass just to take the edge off the day."

Paul was pleased Damien was asking for it. He'd be nice and loose, but coherent, for their little interview. In the beginning, anyway. And then...it wouldn't matter.

"One bowl. No more until after we figure out what we want to do about Joshua. Besides, you don't want to be wasted when we get to that surprise I promised you."

Damien's beady brown eyes lit up. "Do you really have it? Did you really get some for me?"

"For us, not just for you. I want to party too. So, will you fill me in on your good news?"

They passed the pipe. Paul had taken something already to steady his nerves, so he drew the smoke into his lungs lightly. Damien sucked greedily. Watching him, Paul was caught off guard by a fleeting hint of sadness. Instead of Damien Rees, the man sitting in front of him, he saw the cocky little twelve year old who'd never learned how to play. Get rid of that kind of thinking! This was no time to be getting soft about the guy just because he was under a death sentence.

Paul listened intently to Damien's story, especially the proof Damien had uncovered about Joshua's forays into narcotics. It was magnificent. With those details captured on tape, and in C.C.A.'s chief operating officer's own voice, Joshua would have no choice but to agree to whatever proposals Paul presented to him.

Revenge was sweet, but blackmail even sweeter. Paul watched carefully for any openings Damien might give to interject the carefully designed phrases that would help tie his finished recording together. He was thrilled when Damien started ranting about his disdain for Joshua and the other physicians.

"Joshua had the balls to get on my case for the lousy twenty-thousand dollars a year I get paid as a director on Big Blue's board," Damien complained.

"You must've wanted to explode. Our board never wanted to pay you what you were worth."

"Believe me," Damien said, "more than once I've felt like packing it in and letting the bastards try to run the place by themselves. You wouldn't believe what I have to put up with on a daily basis. They treat me like I was a leper. It's more than I can handle sometimes." Damien leaned toward Paul as they sat on the sofa, nearly touching his knee. The more he allowed his feelings to come out in his speech, the closer his body got to Paul's.

Damien was in such an exceptionally vulnerable state. The man's need for affection was so palpable, it was scary.

No. Put aside those feelings. He couldn't afford to feel anything for Damien Rees. His survival depended upon it. Yet he deeply enjoyed the flattery of knowing that Damien was on the verge of admitting his desire for Paul was changing into need. This turned Damien into putty in Paul's hands.

"Damien, this is nothing short of brilliant, your discovery of Joshua's drug habit," Paul egged him on. "I've dreamed for years of ways to make Joshua squirm. Now you've given it to us."

"I've waited, too," Damien said. "He deserves the agony of a slow death. I've thought of a million different ways to pull the plug on him, including handcuffing him to a bed. Oh—" Damien said, "speaking of which, let's take a break. I want to show you the new toys I bought for us."

Okay. He surely had enough material so far to construct a believable set of last words from Damien Rees.

Contingencies ticked away in his brain. Tony, the concierge downstairs, would vouch for Paul's visit to Damien for the evening before Damien's unfortunate and untimely suicide. Paul would later tell the authorities that their work meeting had to be cut short because Damien was feeling depressed and tired.

Remember to take one of Damien's personal envelopes when he left, so that the last words of a devoted senior executive would arrive on Paul's desk tomorrow morning.

"Okay. Show me the toys and then I'll go down to the car and get my surprise."

"I thought you said you had it!" Damien exclaimed angrily.

"The toys won't be any fun without the stuff."

"Cool it. I told you I got it and I do. But I didn't want to raise Tony's suspicion by carrying my little black doctor's bag upstairs to a business meeting. Although, it wouldn't surprise me if he didn't have a pretty good idea what kind of monkey business we get into. He'd be fun to swing with, don't you think?"

Paul touched Damien's knee and started drawing a line up his thigh toward his hips. Damien would be thinking the plan they were developing sounded too good to be true, that they might actually be able to force Joshua to resign. Yes, Paul understood that Machiavellian mind of his. He'd be counting on Paul putting his weight behind Damien as the next president of C.C.A. too.

"Yeah, I'm sorry. It's been a really draining day," Damien said. "You're smart to be cool with Tony. He looks tasty, but I'm not interested in sharing our treats with him or anybody else."

"Me either. Tonight will be our night to remember. Why don't you jump in the shower first? I'll go down to the basement and get my bag of goodies out of the car. Give me your elevator key so I can get back up without Tony having to buzz you again."

Damien's round lips broadened into a grin to that repeated stroke on his thigh. "Good thinking. The keys are on the table by the door. Don't be too long, baby."

"I won't be!" he said, holding his hands out about twelve inches apart. "At least not until I get back up here. And don't you go wasting one in the shower. Save it all for me. Now, show me which keys I need."

"This one works the basement elevator and this one opens the apartment door. Give me a kiss before you go so I'll have something to remember you by while you're gone."

Paul started soft, then put his tongue into Damien's mouth, slowly and lasciviously caressing the inside of his cheeks, his lips and tongue. He waited until Damien started to moan before he pulled out.

"What's the matter? Your memory going? Got the plague? ... Alzheimer's is incurable, you know."

Damien's eyes froze for a split second and Paul cursed himself for the hidden meaning in his words. He laughed, as if he'd said something deliberately stupid, and pursed his lips in an air kiss. Damien turned and headed for the bath.

Paul exited from the lobby so Tony would be sure to see him leaving.

"Going already, Dr. Blake? That was a quickie."

"The boss man is feeling really down. Work is only making him more depressed so we agreed to knock it off for today. He's hitting the sack, so leave the 'Do Not Interruptus' sign on his door."

"Just like the doctor ordered. Have a nice evening."

Paul walked quickly to his car and unlocked the trunk. Opening his black bag, he checked the contents. All the medical paraphernalia he needed was there. The second tape recorder was all set. This was going to be an Academy Award-winning performance, at least among the sadistic aficionados of telephone sex.

He rubbed the back of his neck. He was due for a full-body massage, the stress and tension getting to him. Barring that, a little upper would take care of it. He looked to make sure he had some isobutyl nitrite left in his bag. With any luck, he'd be on his way to the top of the world in less than half an hour.

He opened the basement door to the elevator from the parking lot and went back up to Damien's apartment undetected by Tony. Inside the shower still sloshed. Everything was going according to plan.

First on the agenda was cocaine. Damien would most certainly want a fix, because it was the only way he could relax enough to let Paul give him the yohimbine. When they partied like this, Paul joined Damien in everything. He'd best not change the routine tonight, or Damien's natural paranoia would freak him right out of taking the second injection.

Damien came out of the bathroom drying his balding head to find Paul already with the tourniquet on his arm. "Save some of that for me. Don't you want to shower first?"

The first rush of coke had already stoked Paul's senses. This whole venture was going to be a piece of cake. He could play with it. He might even enjoy it.

"I'll shower after you and I work up a sweat. Get your pretty little ass over here so we can get started."

Damien wiped his crotch one last time and dropped the towel where he stood.

"Okay. I'm coming. At least get undressed first, so I don't feel I'm at a disadvantage. What do you think of the new sheets?"

Damien took a position on the bed to watch Paul undress. Paul took his time, neatly folding every piece as it came off or hanging it on the wooden valet by the clothes closet. Damien was laughing at him, but he didn't care. They were both sticklers for details.

Naked, Paul went to his medical bag and pulled out a new clean needle and a full vial of the liquid elixir. He felt supremely confident, smooth. Damien waited like a sacrificial lamb on his pink sheets, holding out his arm for the needle but looking away. All the better for Paul—making it easy to drain a little extra from the needle into Damien's bulging vein.

Paul ran his hands over the silky coolness of the sheets. "Hrnrnm. Like the skin on a baby's ass. I just hope yours doesn't slip and slide allover the place when I start banging it around."

"Promises, promises. Let's see some action."

"Lay down for a minute so I can get the coke into you. I'll need another minute to prepare our surprise."

The effect of the extra large dose was instantaneous. Damien sat upright on the bed, trying to support his wobbly head. He watched Paul drain the vial with glazed eyes, his tongue hanging out of his mouth loosely. Paul took advantage of his captive audience to extract as much drama from the ritual as possible. He held the needle up and discharged a tiny pearl of the precious aphrodisiac, to make sure there was no air in the needle. Then he sat on the edge of the bed and leaned back slightly, feeling for the pulse beating in his femoral artery deep in his groin.

Then he positioned the razor-sharp tip of the needle at a 45-degree angle to its flow.

"Okay, I'm ready," he said. "Start the countdown."

Damien straightened up. "On your mark. Get set. Go. Ten, nine, eight, seven, six, five … And there she blows!" he squealed. He reached eagerly for Paul's fully erect, engorged penis, stroking it a few times. "My God, I can't believe I'm going to be able to eat the whole thing."

"It's a beauty. Now … it's your turn." Paul gently removed Damien's hand. He took a second vial and a new needle from his bag. "This is a potluck meal. You're not going to get anything to eat until you bring some meat to the table yourself. Lie down so I can get you up and ready too."

Damien gritted his teeth.

"It'll be over in a second, baby. Relax," Paul said.

Damien closed his eyes. "You don't mind if I don't watch?"

"Of course not. It'll only enhance your pleasure when it hits you."

His skilled fingers found Damien's femoral artery, and its parallel vein that carried the blood away from the pelvic area back to the heart. With the sense he was performing a last rite of affection, Paul gently stroked Damien's flaccid penis. It twitched at his touch.

"Ready, Damien?"

Damien took a deep breath. "I'm ready. Let's go."

"When you feel the pin prick and I say go, you can start your own countdown. Count slow. No cheating."

Paul felt carefully again with his fingers. The line between life and death was thin, but he was sure. He penetrated the thin membrane of skin that marked the line and pushed the plunger of the syringe home. "Go."

"Ten, nine, eight, seven, six … "

Damien fell silent.

Very impressive. Paul had to give Damien credit for having the strength to get down to six, which was no easy feat when a double dose of sodium pentathol had been sent streaming up to your heart. It would make an absolutely awesome tape.

Damien lay limp. Paul injected a massive overdose of cocaine into Damien's right arm, the same one as the previous fix. He wiped the syringe clean of his own prints and placed it in Damien's other hand, closing the fingers around the tube and aligning his thumb with the plunger.

Damien was left-handed.

Damien was beginning to convulse as his heart fought for oxygen. Paul suddenly felt very faint. He had ingested a mixture of drugs himself, but the spinning sensation rattling through his head unnerved him. He felt as if he were outside his own body, floating, viewing it in a Kafkaesque scene that unfolded without his volition. He had no capacity to stop it or alter it in any way.

Damien's convulsions were causing his cock to wiggle like a finger, beckoning Paul to come closer. The image mesmerized and revolted him at the same time, so Paul turned Damien onto his stomach so he wouldn't see it. But the sight of Damien's naked buttocks only made him crazier. He fumbled frantically in his bag, hunting for the condom he knew was in there. When he found it, he ripped it open and forced it onto his throbbing cock, hardly conscious of the pain he caused in his haste. He fell onto Damien's body and rammed himself up Damien's ass.

His orgasm began to boil, shaking the words out of him. He heard himself screaming: "You motherfucker! You rotten motherfucker ..."

But something was wrong—very wrong. He grabbed at his heart and collapsed onto Damien.

Twenty-One

Just across the Wisconsin border, the Root River flowed in a torrent. Joshua stood mesmerized, watching the waters wash over
a magnificent steelhead trout that hovered just above its sandy
bottom. The fish's tail barely moved, just enough to keep its
long, sleek body steady against the onrushing current. The trout
glided slowly to the surface. The dorsal fin broke the water's
surface and hesitated, as if the fish had a periscope searching its
surroundings for possible enemies. Then, with a thrusting surge,
it leaped into the sunlight, filling its lungs with air before diving
back down to the safety of its underwater lair.

Joshua was certain the fish had seen him. How could it have
not? He had announced his arrival in a grand manner with a
tremendous crashing noise when he slipped and almost fell into
the river. He cursed himself loudly for his clumsiness, and the
sound of his voice had echoed through the silence of the forest
like a roll of thunder. A half bottle of Jack Daniels had conspired
with the slippery rocks dotting the river's edge to dump him
into the water, and now he seriously wondered if he could stay
dry long enough to catch that trophy-sized beauty quivering a
few yards away.

When he first saw the trout, he could hardly believe its size.
Water always magnified the size of submerged objects, but this
was not an average-sized fish. It was colossal. In the clamor of

Joshua's arrival, the fish had turned tail and shot like a missile for the safety of a fallen tree that lay under the ledge of the far bank, leaving behind a swirl that sucked small branches flowing by into a gaping vortex.

Trophies didn't grow to that size by being stupid or impatient. Joshua would have to sit very quietly for a good long while before casting his line. He'd probably have to wait until the last light of day before the giant fish could be lured again.

Physically and emotionally drained, he'd promised himself to lay off his drugs until Ruth's operation and the C.C.A. crisis had blown over, but no way would he be able to match the patience of the trout with his nerves in their current shape. So just this once more, he told himself, as he popped a few uppers and laid his fly rod up against a nearby log on the riverbank.

Exhaustion, alcohol, and the pills might make him doze off. So he set his watch alarm for thirty minutes. Night would be falling by then, and the river would take on a glassy smoothness to reflect a full moon already emerging in the sky overhead. Joshua regarded it through the chemical mist clouding his mind. That arrogant monster hiding itself across the pool would soon be his.

He laid his head back on a clump of grass on the bank. His eyes closed. The barrier between waking and sleeping dreams, the twilight zone before a blackout, dissolved and Joshua slid seamlessly into a deeper dream.

"A fine kettle of fish you've gotten yourself into, Joshua."

How many years since he'd heard the sarcastic tone of his father's voice? The shock of its familiarity thrust him back to the brink of consciousness.

"Who's that? Who's that talking?"

"Don't play games with me, Joshua. You've been ignoring me for years and look where it's gotten you."

Was he speaking out loud? He couldn't break through the gauze curtain that had settled over his mind. His father's voice

---

290

was louder than the rushing roar of the river at his feet. Had his father actually died, or did Joshua only dream that his childhood wishes had come true and finally eliminated his father's tormenting scrutiny of his everyday life?

"I can take care of myself. I don't need any help, especially from you."

His father's laugh was sinister. "Oh, you can, can you? Not very well, as far as I can tell!"

Joshua rolled over heavily and pushed himself up to a sitting position by sheer force of will. His head felt like lead. If he could just get up and walk to the river's edge, feel the cold water on his hands and face, he'd wake up.

At the river's edge he bent down on one knee and reached into the cold water, cupped a handful and splashed it onto his face. When he shook the water out of his eyes, he looked up to see Martin Caliban sitting on the log beside Joshua's fly rod, just behind the clump of grass where Joshua had put his head down. He looked as solid as a rock, but surely he was no more than a chimera created by fatigue and worry and drugs. Just a bad trip and nothing more.

"You'll never get me out of your blood, out of your genes."

Joshua sank to his knees, continuing to shake his head, but the vision wouldn't clear. "What do you want from me? I've got enough to handle without having to deal with you. And for God's sake, don't sit on my rod. It's my favorite."

Martin Caliban sat back down on the log. He caressed the rod with what seemed genuine admiration. Then he gently moved it to a boulder next to him. "I ain't going to break it. It's a beaut. Graphite, isn't it? In our day, everything was split bamboo. We didn't have this fancy stuff."

Joshua felt faint. How many years of his life had he waited to hear such words of admiration from Martin Caliban? Now, here in front of him, a man who looked like his father and sounded

291

like him was admiring Joshua's fishing rod. Joshua imagined the hand caressing the rod running down the back of his own taut neck.

"What do you want from me, Dad? I've got a lot of things on my mind."

Martin stroked the rod once again, gently, tenderly. The tension in Joshua's neck let go ever so slightly. "Actually, you may not believe this, but I just want to help."

Was this *his* father? Was this concern without a trace of condescension or self-righteousness really coming from his father's heart? Martin had offered help many times before, but it had never come without a price attached. Joshua was too practiced at protecting himself from the hidden barbs in his father's peace offerings to take this new twist at face value.

"Sure! Sure! Like you helped when I was growing up. Haven't you done enough damage already?"

Martin's bushy brown eyebrows drooped, his thick full lips sagged at the corners. Was that sadness Joshua saw? The Martin Caliban Joshua had known never had admitted he felt misunderstood, had always tried to defend and win a point, had never explained and clarified his thoughts or actions. Martin's aim had always been to induce guilt and shame, never to give his son solace.

"My life wasn't peaches and cream, you know," his father continued. "When you were fourteen years old, I took you fishing on this river. When I was fourteen years old, I had no time to fish. Don't you talk to me about damage. 'Hard Knocks' was the only university I could attend. If I didn't work, my mother and sisters didn't eat. I had to take care of them."

"If that's the case, what's the difference now, Dad? What's softened you up?" Joshua felt cheated that his father now should begin to turn into a human being.

"You don't know what happens after death, Joshua. Let's just say I've had more education since I left this world."

Joshua stood up. For a split second he toyed with the idea of bending over and picking up the big rock sitting next to his foot and heaving it at this phantom. He would shatter the image that had tormented him once and for all. But he squared off in front of Martin instead.

"Too bad we couldn't take advantage of your wisdom earlier," he spat. "I'll just bet you took better care of Grandma than you did of Mom! Did you treat your mistresses the same way you did Mom? Did you beat them up when they didn't please you? I still carry the stripes of your 'caring' to this day. Don't think I'll ever forget it."

The look of sadness on his father's face dissolved into one of such deep anguish and pain it took Joshua completely by surprise. He could never have imagined seeing such an expression from this man. The Martin Caliban he remembered had ice water running in his veins, colder than the melted snow flowing in the river behind him.

"There are some things maybe you'll never be able to understand about your mother, Joshua. And especially about your mother and me. It was your mother's depression that killed her spirit and her will to live, long before cancer took her life. But she was a very understanding woman. We had an unspoken agreement about other women. We did what we had to do to keep our relationship intact. You have no right to judge us, or anyone else."

Joshua was speechless, quaking with indignation. He raised his hand, pointed a menacing finger at the image before him and shook it. Memories of his own past dalliances with O.R. nurses flickered like the shadows of an old reel of film across his mind. But they faded quickly only to be replaced by the terror he had seen on Ruth's face the night he threatened to hit her in his rage. His confusion made him even angrier.

"Depression didn't kill Mom! Stopping the IV feeding her did! And you didn't even have the fucking guts to pull the plug yourself!" He almost choked on his words. He sputtered to a stop and listened to the breath rasping in his throat as if it belonged to someone else. It burned all the way up from his bowels. His pulse raced. Joshua rubbed his chest just below his heart, but it did nothing to ease the dreadful ache. The sweat stood out on his forehead and ran down his face in streams. It couldn't be. His father was wiping tears from his eyes. He'd seen his father cry only once, when his mother died.

"I'm sorry for having done that to you. I felt so guilty for all the shit I'd put her through. I just couldn't bring myself to be responsible."

"No! No!" Joshua fell to his knees and collapsed, sobbing quietly. "What about ... what about the empty ... the empty safe deposit box?"

Martin looked down at his feet. "I was too ... too ashamed, too proud, to tell you I had spent it all. I...."

"Spent it! Don't lie to me!" Joshua was on his feet again, his temper throbbing with adrenaline. "Hell, you gambled it away! You were addicted to the ponies!"

"Yes, I did have a gambling problem. But ... oh hell, I guess it doesn't make any damn difference now! A ton of unpaid medical bills. Your medical school tuition. Those were my burdens. I had no choice. Sure, you had pain and suffering. But at least you had Ruth to help. Who did I have to lean on?"

Joshua shook. "You're damn right! It doesn't make any difference. It's too late to take away the pain. You can't apologize for a lifetime of hurt."

His father was moving toward him, his short stocky arms reaching out as if to hug him. Joshua took a step backwards and held up his right hand to stop him. The figure stood still and hung its head.

"What is it you wanted from me, Joshua? What could I have done differently?"

"You could've loved me. That's all I really ever wanted." Joshua could hardly speak through his tears.

"I loved you the only way I knew how. I still love you and I always will. You're my flesh and blood. You are my dearest son."

The words ricocheted inside Joshua's mind, fighting to fend off the insistent wristwatch alarm trying to invade his dream. He couldn't decide whether he desperately wanted this horrible nightmare to end, or if he wanted to stay asleep and work through the questions tormenting his mind.

How could his father have changed so much after death, finally saying the things he should have spoken in life? Had everything he suffered in his childhood just been some kind of bad joke? And now, was he supposed to forgive this man? Did he even want to?"Well, it wasn't good enough. You could've done a hell of a lot better."

Martin rubbed his bald head. "For your sake, stop hating me. Let go of your anger, or it will poison you." Martin's voice was starting to fade. The alarm was winning the battle.

Joshua pushed off his watch alarm. He looked around at the empty bank and heard the river's voice endlessly repeating itself behind him. What was he doing standing up? Hadn't he just lain down? The skies were clear, but a small shower must have passed by to explain the dampness on his face. He'd been dreaming. It seemed important, as if something of great significance had happened, but try as he might, his conscious mind couldn't recapture the vague thread of its meaning.

And, he could have sworn that he'd left his rod leaning up against the log, not the boulder where it now lay. No matter, he'd found it. And that trout was still waiting for him.

Joshua reached for the black spider lure he kept in one of his vest pockets. Still groggy, he recoiled slightly from touching it. He had a thing about spiders. Some weeks ago, in a fit of temper, he'd tried to rid the garage of all the spiders nesting in there. Ruth was openly dismayed at the intensity of his anger, and pulled out one of her books on symbols and read to him a passage on the creatures.

Spiders, she said, often symbolized the unending cycle of life and death. A spider's constant building up and tearing down illustrates our life-long processes of transmutation. Even as the thread of an old life ended in death, it was already being spun again into a new pattern. Native Americans believed that a spider woman sings the universe into being as she spins. Why was he reminded of this passage now? Why was it resonating so oddly with his soul? It felt familiar, like something that may have happened in his dream moments before.

Joshua shrugged it off and attended to his fly line, his practiced fingers working smoothly. His heart started to pound the second he stepped in the water. The moon was high now. Squinting, he tried to catch a glint of light reflecting off the scales of the fish lying across the stream behind the submerged log. He didn't see anything, but it didn't daunt his expectations in the least. He could feel the giant's presence in his nerves. It would probably tip the scales at several pounds. Maybe it was even big enough to replace the trophy hanging in his office, the one that was only a pound shy of his father's best record.

Joshua tried to relax. His presentation would have to be flawless to get the fish's attention without raising an alarm. He would have to be skillful enough to make it seem that the spider had just fallen from the tree above, struggling to grab hold of something.

Joshua knew this particular stretch of river very well. He and his father had fished it from the time Joshua was a teenager. The water's smooth and glassy surface even though it was racing by at a constant speed had always intrigued him. The river was constantly changing, but this was really only noticeable when the speed of the flow shifted, or when something like a tree fell in to dam its progress. It was always a crisis that defined movement.

The moon overhead seemed extraordinarily bright, perhaps because the night sky was so clear and the stars had no competition from city lights. The racing river lulled him. He couldn't be sure if he were standing on the shore looking at a reflection on the water, or floating on the water looking at a reflection of the shore.

The moon shone on his face. That would make his silhouette less visible to the trout prowling beneath the surface a few yards away. The moment came and he made his cast automatically, without thinking. The eight-foot graphite pole slipped easily through the air as if it were his scalpel, a part of his arm.

A picture book cast. The fly line landed first, settling gently on the water some twenty feet upstream. The tapered leader line and delicate trace swooped in right behind. The spider landed on the water with not a ripple more than the real thing would have made, and the moving water caused its hairy legs to wiggle in front of the fish's nose.

Before Joshua's conscious mind had even registered any movement in the water, he felt his wrist instinctively stiffen. The huge creature had made a swirling vortex with its tail to suck in the spider, but had failed. They would both have to try again. Joshua resigned himself to patience, emulating his quarry. He retrieved the fly and checked it to make sure it wasn't marred. Satisfied that it was still in perfect shape and that the point of the hook was razor sharp, Joshua steeled himself for a second cast.

His heart was beating as fast as it did at the climax of making love. He had to make himself stand still, breathing deeply, until

---

he could gaze at the glistening wavelets on the moonlit river without trembling. He stripped the line off of his reel, then slowly knelt to scoop up some water onto his face. The night sounds receded and all his movements shifted downward into a smooth, elongated sequence. He was concentrating so hard he was barely aware of what he did, and yet, at the same time, his focus seemed strangely magnified.

He watched the spider creeping in slow motion along the length of the submerged log. Joshua had arrived at the heart of the magic—that place where driving obsession arises. The very instant he recognized the obsession, he let it go. He knew that uncontrolled zeal would cause him to push too hard and would cost him his trophy. Landing this wily opponent would take subtle finesse, a balance between pushing and pulling.

The fountain of molten silver that sprayed in the moonlight shattered his philosophical musing. It had to be only his imagination, but he could have sworn he saw the pink throat of the fish as it tried to swallow the entire river in one gulp. He counted to three before setting the hook, but it seemed more like three hundred. Just as the number burst from his lips, the trout crashed back into the river with such force that its own thrashing pulled the point through the tough gristle at the corner of its jaw. The battle was on.

Joshua's job now was to hang onto the trampolining fish and pray that its will to escape upstream would run out before the line that was smoking off of his reel melted. The trout reversed its direction. It must have sensed it was using too much energy going against the current. It torpedoed downstream.

Sweat poured from Joshua. This was a dangerous point. If the fish persevered in this way, the combination of its own strength and the natural force of the river would mean inevitable escape. Joshua had no choice. He scurried along the slippery rocks to keep up with the mighty fish.

In his excitement and still inebriated state, he stumbled in the shallow water at the river's edge.

"Shit! Fuck!" Blood dripped from a gash on the palm of the hand he'd used to break his fall. But the instant Joshua felt the throbbing pressure of the trout still attached to his line, he forgot about the pain.

He looked down at the face of his reel and its backing in dismay. If he lost any more line, the battle was over. He would have to take a gamble. He pointed the tip of the rod to the galaxies and sent a series of sharp; punching jabs down the vibrating line, the kind a boxer would deliver to weaken an opponent.

A surge of pleasure coursed through him. He was shifting the pain in his wrist to the fish's jaw. "How about a little of your own medicine, you bastard!"

It was as if the fish heard him. The trout stopped and turned defiantly to face its attacker, then sank to the bottom of the river like a stone.

A brief standoff. Enough time for both opponents to catch their breaths. Joshua's most immediate task was to regain some line. Since the fish wasn't about to give it back, Joshua would have to go get it. He started to move slowly downstream. "Okay, if the mountain won't come to Mohammed, Mohammed will go to the mountain," he muttered.

The line slackened slightly, and the fish rested for a few more seconds before launching another powerful rush upstream. It exploded out of the water in an acrobatic leap of energy and beauty right in front of his face. For a second, he actually thought he saw the trout smile broadly, but he didn't have the strength to return the greeting. He found himself working prodigiously to keep up.

If at any time the fish decided to turn and make a committed run downstream without stopping, the contest would be over. Joshua would never be able to close the gap between them, no matter how fast he ran. Joshua had a sudden hallucinatory notion that he was the prey, that the fish that was playing him at the end of the line and not the other way around.

But all thoughts faded as his entire consciousness was consumed with staying on his feet, keeping the line straight and not falling behind and losing distance. No feeling of exhaustion or pain.

Only the will to win remained. He lost count of the number of times the fish led him back and forth, up and down the river. He became vaguely aware of a warmth seeping down his legs from his groin. He'd urinated in his boots. His arms ached fiercely from holding the end of the rod high up in the air.

Suddenly he realized he wasn't moving. The trout sulked. Joshua's heart skipped a beat. The water dimpled as if the fish were preparing to leap out. But instead of its massive silver body silhouetted against the black river, only its giant head broke the surface. The river's current erased the few ripples.

The fish's spirit was nearly broken. A few more bouts of racing up and downstream, or flat-out desperate runs for freedom, but the battle was over. Only a matter of time before the fish would be his. Time to be careful.

"Come to me, baby. Come to Papa," Joshua panted with exhaustion.

But his excitement started to grow again. The trout was strong. It had fought well and with intelligence. Joshua's arms felt as if he'd been pulling the entire river bottom up along with the trout for the last twenty yards. Joshua admired the fact that the fish couldn't be wrenched from its place. It would only be taken by patience. Draw the trout to him inch by inch. Stay alert.

He licked some of the sweat that had gathered along his upper lip. His tongue felt like a sponge left out in the sun. He thought fondly about the bottle of bourbon he'd left back in the cabin, but forgot about it in the next second as he got his first good look at the trout. Its last thrust up into the air revealed a creature fully fifty percent bigger than the biggest fish his father had ever dreamed of landing.

"Jesus! Jesus Christ! Wait till Ruth sees this baby hanging in the office!"

Joshua focused. A dozen more careful turns of the reel. Then the dream of a lifetime lay helplessly before his feet. He stood over his vanquished foe, elated beyond words. A white eye stared back up, reflecting the moon like a searchlight. The fish waited patiently for Joshua's next move, just as it had in the water. Its gills pumped oxygen rhythmically.

Joshua watched the eye. No answering emotion of any kind. Only a pinpoint of light. Unwavering. Undimmed. He stared at it until he lost his point of reference again, hypnotized, the sensation of one watching himself as a detached observer. His left hand, the injured one, grabbed the fish's lower jaw between his thumb and second finger. Blood beaded out of his fingers, punctured by the trout's sharp teeth. With his other hand, he reached down to remove the spider lure.

It fell away without his touching it. Joshua instinctively gripped a little harder. The trout had no fear of death. It made no struggle. Joshua fumbled at his fishing vest for the small wooden club.

"Shit!"

He couldn't disfigure a fish to be mounted as a trophy by hitting it on the head. He dropped the club. Still moving as if outside himself, Joshua reached under his vest to a pocket in the shirt he'd worn straight from the office. He found a pencil that weighed heavier in his hand than a scalpel. He held it poised, pointing at the fish's eye as it looked up at him. He couldn't move. His hand was frozen in midair, as still as death.

Death. Joshua shuddered and time began to move again. He was about to sign another death certificate. His vision went dark. A cloud had suddenly appeared, briefly covering the face of the moon. The fish's eye still gleamed like the glow of phosphorescent plankton in a sea of black ink.

He threw the pencil into the river and watched it float around and around in an eddy at his feet before it disappeared into the darkness. Joshua released his grip on the trout's jaw. He gently cradled the fish in both of his hands. It lay heavy and substantial, quiescent, yet still pulsing with life. It was something beautiful, imbued with spirit … and no longer his adversary. A growing joy crept into the edge of his thoughts.

Joshua rocked the trout back and forth in the water like an infant in its first bath, willing strength back into it. He didn't need to push it away. With a regal stateliness, the fish simply glided off into the current.

Joshua walked back to the cabin with a quiet mind. His skin felt cool where the sweat had dried in the breeze. The ache in his legs and his wrist were like badges of honor, his battle wounds. This quiet elation was new to him. It was like the stillness and exhaustion that follow birth wrapping around him like a receiving blanket.

Inside the cabin, he downed half of what was left of the Jack Daniels in one swig. He stripped off his sweat-soaked, urine-stained boots and clothes and washed down two halcyon pills with the rest of the bourbon, a knockout punch if there ever was one. No dreams would disturb his sleep tonight.

He set his watch alarm for four-thirty. That would give him enough time to be back at the hospital by seven a.m. Joshua unstrapped the watch from his badly bruised wrist. He could hardly believe his eyes. He'd hooked the fish at dusk, which was at about nine p.m., and here it was almost quarter to midnight.

Twenty-Two

Mary glanced over her bifocals at the clock and shook her head. Seven-thirty a.m. Was it an omen? If so, today could make yesterday's hell look like a vacation. Peter, noticeably upset, called to see if she'd heard from Joshua who was already late for their breakfast meeting. If he didn't arrive soon, he'd miss seeing Ruth before she went into surgery. Mary immediately tried to reach Joshua on his pager and car phone, to no avail. They were out of range. She'd even tried the phone in Peter's cabin, letting it ring several times before hanging up.

Mary had been through days like this before. Meal breaks would be few and far between, so the soft-boiled eggs cooking on the hot plate in Joshua's office might be the only hot meal she'd get for a while. She looked down at the hourglass on her desk. The grains of sand in the upper half were jockeying for position. When the last one had made its way through the opening, time would be up. Time was shifting too, standing still for no one, not even for Joshua Caliban. The instant she saw the light flashing on Joshua's private line, Mary turned the heat off under the pot. Her hot, three-minute egg was going to be cold and hard-boiled.

"Good morning. Dr. Caliban's office."

"Mary. It's me. I need you to make a few phone calls."

Not even "hello." This told her all she needed to know about Joshua's frame of mind. The sun may have been shining outside, but it was going to be a dark day inside C.C.A.

"Are you all right, Dr. Caliban? Dr. Albert has been trying to reach you."

"He's the first one I need to talk to. I'll hold on while you page him. When you find him, patch me through."

"Certainly, Dr. Caliban."

Looking up at the clock, she decided to gamble on calling the O.R. first.

"Kathy," she said, "this is Mary. Dr. Caliban is urgently trying to reach Dr. Albert."

"He's about to begin operating on Ruth. Hang on a second."

Half consciously, Mary turned the three-minute hourglass back over. The grains of sand moved like frozen molasses.

"Mary, Dr. Albert says to tell Dr. Caliban that he's begun the surgery and can't be interrupted. He also wants you to try to track down Dr. Blake. Dr. Blake never showed up this morning for surgery, or called in."

"Not a happy trooper this morning, I gather."

"You've got that right. Later."

If Peter Albert wasn't a happy trooper, Joshua was going to be a miserable general. Mary had a sick feeling she knew why Joshua wasn't here for his wife's operation. The sands were emptying the hourglass rapidly. Joshua himself would soon slip through the vortex and have to stop running. Mary decided Joshua didn't need to know about Dr. Blake's absence at this moment.

"Dr. Caliban. Sorry to keep you waiting. Dr. Albert has begun Mrs. Caliban's surgery already and cannot be interrupted."

"Shit! Damn! There' s no fucking way. ..."

Mary winced.

"I'll be back by nine-thirty, ten at the latest," Joshua said, after a protracted silence. "Please ask Jane to schedule a meeting at four this afternoon in the boardroom. I want Polanski, Carter, and Jackson to be there. Oh yeah, she'd better include Simple Simmons. Tell her it's absolutely vital that they be there. You'll need to organize an emergency board meeting for one today. I'll explain everything then. If Moerae is available, please be sure she's at the meeting as well."

"What about Mr. Rees?" Mary thought she knew the answer, but these days she took nothing for granted.

"Absolutely not. In fact, he shouldn't even be around these days. I told him to take some vacation until further notice."

"I'll take care of it all. And … please drive carefully."

"You'll be able to get me on my car phone in about an hour if you need me. See you soon."

As she hung up the phone, Mary leaned back in her chair and rubbed her hands. No rain in sight. Was her arthritis sensing the storm brewing at C.C.A.? Would Joshua survive his battle? And Ruth hers?

The last few grains of sand were falling through the waist in her hourglass. She plucked the pencil she kept in her bun by her ear and stuck it between her teeth. It helped her think, and she needed to collect her thoughts to develop a plan of attack.

The board meeting would be the easiest to schedule. It was the power brokers' meeting that was more unusual, so she'd start with that one and then try to locate the elusive Dr. Blake. Leaning forward, she dialed the first number.

"Hello Liz, Mary. Is your boss in yet?"

"Hi, Mary. No. She was burning the midnight oil. Has today's flood begun already?"

"Like Montezuma's revenge," Mary answered." It's urgent that I speak with her. Can you track her down?"

"Give me fifteen minutes. Keep me plugged in if I can help."

Mary looked up as Elaine MacDonald sauntered into her office, a plastic smile painted across her heavily made-up face. The last thing Mary needed this morning was to waste time being polite to a doctor's wife, especially one she detested. Mary Howard could tolerate most people, but Elaine was one of the few exceptions.

"Hi, Elaine. Grab a cup. I'll be right with you. I've got an urgent call to make."

"Don't let me interfere. I just dropped by to see Ruth but I missed her. The traffic was terrible this morning, wasn't it?"

Mary turned to look up the next number. Elaine seldom lied outright. Usually she told only the part of the truth that suited her purpose. If she'd missed seeing Ruth, it had nothing to do with the traffic.

Mary had first tried Paul's home number and left a message on his answering machine asking him to call her office. She was now ringing a second number, a friend's who worked as a security Guard at Paul's apartment. "Sarah. Hi. This is Mary. Listen, I haven't got time to schmooze right now. I'm trying to track down Dr. Blake. Would you have any idea what time he left his apartment this morning?"

Mary's squared chin dropped when Sarah informed her that as far as she could tell Paul Blake hadn't come home last night. No way Elaine's watchful eyes missed the surprise on her face. Sarah explained briefly. She was certain because his little red Porsche wasn't in its parking space as of three a.m.

"Thanks, Sarah. If you happen to see him, would you please have him call Dr. Caliban's office immediately? Yeah, let's do lunch soon."

Elaine's prominent nose was twitching and her rouged cheeks wrinkled. Mary said, "Those guys will do anything to avoid being called in for special board meetings. I've got to call the rest of the board. What can I do for you?"

"Just a quickie. I'm planning a surprise party for Scottie and I don't want the invitations floating around here. I've misplaced Damien's home address. You wouldn't have it by any chance, would you?"

The bright smile Elaine flashed didn't fool Mary for a second, but she had more important things to do right then than entertain Elaine's dalliances. Most importantly, she didn't need Elaine's big ears and bigger nose hanging around. Mary spun her Rolodex. She knew that if she acted like Elaine was one of the girls, it would be easier to manipulate her into leaving quickly.

"I'm pretty sure it's where the bigwigs live over at Lakeshore Tower North. Yes, here it is," she said, copying the exact address on a piece of paper.

"Anything else I can do? I've got a lot of stuff I've got to get done."

Elaine smiled again, but Mary knew it wasn't a sign of thanks. "I'm out of your hair. Thanks for the java and the info. Give Ruth a hug for me if you see her before I do."

Mary would certainly give Ruth a big hug, but not one with Elaine's name on it. Waving a perfunctory good-bye, Mary reached for the red light blinking on Joshua's private line.

"Good morning. Dr. Caliban's office."

"Doesn't sound like it's going to be a good one. Hi, Mary. It's Jane. Liz just called. I didn't get in until almost three this morning."

"Sorry to bother you Jane, but Joshua wants you to organize a power brokers' meeting for four this afternoon in his office."

"Sounds like the battle is heating up. Getting those turkeys into the same room on such short notice won't be easy. I'll need to give them some explanation. Can I speak to Joshua for a second?"

Mary paused. What should she say? Not in or unavailable at the moment were worlds apart. If Joshua wasn't in the building, Jane would know it meant he wasn't there for Ruth before she went into surgery. She wasn't sure whether to lie outright or give Jane just a partial truth.

"He's not in yet. I can have him call you as soon as he arrives."

Jane paused a long moment, and then sighed heavily. "No problem. I'll make sure they're there. Anything else?"

Mary flipped back through the rapidly filling pad on her clipboard. "Oh, yeah. He said if it were possible he wanted to have Moerae attend the board meeting."

"No sweat. She's here now. We've been having a breakfast skull session on the LaPorte suit. I'll make sure she's there, too. We'll be on our way in as soon as I can start the first round of telephone tag. Liz can track me down if you need me. I owe you a hug."

"Thanks, Jane. I could use it."

Sitting in the back of the taxi, Elaine was steaming. When she'd called Paul at his business meeting last night, the voice on the answering machine was familiar, but she hadn't been able to place it at first. Then when Scott had gotten home and started in on his incessant bitching, the light bulb had gone on. She had laid awake the rest of the night telling herself Paul would have a good reason why he and Damien had to meet. The information she'd weaseled out of Damien's secretary this morning that he was taking vacation leave was confusing. Why hadn't Paul just told her the truth?

As soon as she'd been able to get Scott out of the house this morning, she'd tried unsuccessfully to reach Paul at his apartment, on his pager, and at his office. The nurse told her she had no idea where Paul was and that Dr. Albert was fit to be tied. Paul was never late for surgery. Mary's call to Paul's apartment and her attempts to hide her surprise at whatever she'd been told had been the last straw. Mary had probably seen through the lie Elaine told her to get Damien's unlisted home address, but that was of no real consequence. Something smelled fishy and despite her sexual attraction to Paul, she relished the thought of catching her domineering lover with his pants down for once.

Elaine knocked hard on Damien's door several times. No response. A pungent odor like a backed-up toilet seeped out into the hallway. The silence in the apartment triggered a faint wave of panic—she fought to keep it under control. Throwing caution entirely to the wind, she decided to get help.

Tony frowned at the thought of disturbing one of his most finicky tenants. Nevertheless, he returned to Damien's apartment and pounded hard on the substantial door. Worn down by Elaine, he reluctantly reached for his master key. Elaine grabbed Tony's arm as the deadbolt lock clicked open and they entered the living room together.

"Mr. Rees. Mr. Rees, are you home, sir?" Tony called out.

Elaine let out a low gasp, tugged his arm, and motioned toward Damien's half-opened bedroom door. She had caught glimpse of the reflection in the ceiling mirror. She pushed Tony toward the bedroom. A pile of crumpled clothes caught the edge of the door, and Tony had to shove hard.

Tony and Elaine stumbled into the room together. The grisly scene that greeted them stopped them in their tracks.

Damien's nude body was lying prone on his bed, his head turned to the side, showing his mouth agape in frozen horror. Paul's body was stacked atop of Damien's, with his arms draped over Damien's shoulders. Lines of dried blood from his closed eyes striped his sallow cheek.

Her scream filled the room, and most of the next floor down, too.

Twenty-Three

When Mary called saying Joshua had arrived smelling like a subway john and looking like death warmed over, Peter came rushing over. "He won't win any fashion awards," he said to her, holding up a set of surgical greens complete with tie on booties, "but at least I know these'll fit him. Give us a few minutes alone, if you can."

Mary rubbed her temples. "How … how's Ruth?"

Peter smiled and gave her a thumbs-up. "God was with us. I think she's going to be all right. How's Joshua doing?"

"He's just getting out of the shower. I think he's at the end of his rope."

Peter nodded and closed Joshua's office door. Joshua was drying himself when Peter knocked on the bathroom door.

"Is that you, Peter?"

Peter glanced at the pile of clothing crumpled on the floor. "Yeah. I've got something for you to cover your ass, at least temporarily."

"Thanks. Hand it in to me, will you? And there should be a cup of coffee on the credenza, too. I'll be right out."

Although it was good sized, he'd had to remove only a lump, not Ruth's whole breast. As a result, Peter was feeling more compassionate and tolerant than angry toward Joshua who would have to be feeling as guilty as sin. There was no bite to the humor he used to try to take the edge off the moment.

"Yes, massah. Here dey is and da bwana said to tell you dat your missus is gonna be fine."

Except for the grey lines under his bloodshot eyes when Joshua emerged from the bathroom, he looked like a brand new resident wearing his surgical greens for the first time. His eyes flickered awkwardly as they met Peter's for a split second. Peter correctly sensed that a longer glimpse would have produced tears of relief streaming down Joshua's face.

"Thank you, Peter. Tell the bwana he's a better doctor than a haberdasher. When can I see her?"

"She'll be under for at least a couple of hours. They'll call as soon as she starts to stir. Ross has it under his scope now. Only time will tell, but I think it was a clean cut."

"How much did you have to cut?"

"Only a lump."

"Good. Then let's get down to the business at hand. While I was fishing, I had a brainstorm about how to handle the LaPorte suit. What … "

Peter held up his hand. "Please sit down, Joshua. We need to talk, and not about the business stuff. Not yet, anyway. I need an explanation as to why you weren't here this morning. "

Joshua sat down and kicked his desk drawer closed. "Come on, Peter. I'm sorry I stood you up. I got stuck in traffic. I'll pay my breakfast bill, don't worry."

Peter remained standing. No sitting down for this one. "Joshua, I know bullshit when I hear it, and piss when I smell it!" He nodded toward the pile of clothes. "It's time you came clean with me. No half-truths. No missing pieces. What happened last night?"

Joshua's broad shoulders sagged. Peter felt a wave of hope rush through his heart. For as long as he'd known him, Joshua had dealt with pain by forgetting it, putting it out of his mind. Would he finally surrender?

"It sounds like there's an 'or else' at the end of that question, " Joshua said. Peter looked down at Joshua. Usually the man in the green suit was the one standing and the one sitting was being given the final prognosis. He looked Joshua squarely in the eye.

"Or else the day I discharge Ruth from this hospital is the day I discharge myself as well." Peter paused and then finally added, "Waiting won't make it any easier," he said softly.

Joshua leaned forward and began by recounting the story of the fish. He looked down at his wrist." If I hadn't broken my damn watch trying to land that fish, I'd have made it here in time for Ruth."

Peter took a few paces, turned, and caught Joshua's gaze. "Were you already on the road when Mary called the cabin this morning?"

Joshua looked down at the floor. "Actually, I think I was still at the cabin. I'd passed out last night and was still pretty groggy. By the time I got to the phone, she'd hung up. Between the clock on the kitchen wall and the sun streaming through the window, it didn't take a rocket scientist to figure out what had happened." Like the trout he battled the night before, Joshua had no more energy to run away. He began to surrender the truth.

Peter nodded. Each time Joshua hesitated over something painful, Peter simply folded his hands and continued pacing, using the pressure of silence as his prod. Ten minutes later, Joshua finished.

Peter stopped pacing, sat beside Joshua, and locked his hands behind his head. He wasn't so naive as to believe that Joshua had told him everything that had transpired in the last fourteen hours, but he was confident Joshua had told him more of the truth than he'd ever done before.

———

"Well, that's a nice smorgasbord of stuff. What have you taken since you got back?"

Shadows flooded the grayed pools of Joshua's eyes. "Why is that important, Doctor?"

Peter took a deep breath and released it. He would have to be patient. Joshua had to make the decision to ask for help on his own. "I intend to prescribe something to help ease your withdrawal pains. You, of course, are free to seek a second opinion."

Joshua sat without speaking for a moment, finally breaking the silence with a deep sigh. He glanced at his desk drawer. "I just took two dexymyl with my coffee."

Peter reached for the prescription pad on Joshua's desk and scribbled something on it. "Could you please buzz Mary for me? I'll ask her to take this down to pharmacy right away."

"Boy, you don't waste any time, do you, Doc?" He reached for his intercom. "Mary, could you please come in for a second?"

Peter leaned across and placed his right hand on Joshua's shoulder. "'To everything there is a season,' my friend. I think perhaps now it's a time to heal."

Mary came into the office. "Yes, Dr. Caliban."

Peter handed her the prescription. "Could you please ask pharmacy to fill this right away and bring it back up."

Mary took the prescription and clipped it to the top of her ever-present clipboard. "Certainly, Dr. Albert." She turned to Joshua.

Joshua looked down at his bare left wrist, then stole a glance at the clock on his desk. "How are you doing getting everybody together for the board meeting?" he finally said. "And how's it going with the power brokers' meeting?"

"Jane called a few minutes ago. She said curiosity got the cat. They'll all be there. I've been able to get in touch with everyone for the board meeting except Dr. Blake. If you'll give me the keys to your house, I'll have someone pick you up a set of clothes first thing this afternoon."

Joshua smiled broadly. As he scribbled the alarm system code number on a piece of paper, Joshua caught a glimpse of someone entering Mary's outer office. They were wearing uniforms, but they weren't hospital security guards. Two members of the Chicago Police Department were approaching Joshua's door, one male, one female.

"Excuse me for interrupting. Is this Dr. Caliban's office?"

Mary moved toward the two officers, so that she was standing between them and Joshua.

"Yes, it is. How can I help you?"

"We're from the CPD, ma'am," the man said, flipping open his badge.

"It's very urgent that we speak with Dr. Caliban."

"I'm Dr. Caliban. What's the problem, officer?"

He smiled and held out his weathered hand. "Captain Wong, CPD, sir. And this is Detective Roberts," Wong added, nodding toward his partner.

"We're in the midst of several crises, Captain. What can we do for you?"

The captain's eyes studied Joshua and then quickly darted to the crumpled pile of discarded clothes by the bathroom door. "If you have an emergency, Dr. Caliban, we'll just wait."

Joshua shook his head. "No, no. Please be seated. Mary, could you please close the door as you leave and hold all calls except emergencies."

"Certainly, Dr. Caliban." Mary closed the office door behind her.

"I'm afraid we've got some very bad news, Dr. Caliban," Captain Wong said, looking in Peter's direction.

"You can feel perfectly free to speak in front of Dr. Albert," Joshua told him.

For the next ten minutes Peter and Joshua listened in shock. An icy chill shot through the back of Joshua's neck.

"Captain Wong, we are accustomed to blood and guts around here, but your description of what the police found when they arrived sounds absolutely gruesome."

"Ditto," Peter said.

Joshua couldn't believe his ears. He was also having a difficult time reconciling the rattling voices warring again inside his head. Damien's and Paul's grotesque demise had wiped away more than one enormous problem. He might not have to give it up after all. Part of him felt remorse as well. While it hadn't been Joshua's hand that delivered the final blow, he wasn't free of all responsibility for their deaths.

"How is Mrs. MacDonald?" Peter asked.

"She was pretty shaken," Detective Roberts answered. "We convinced her to come along with us to the hospital so they could give her something to calm her down. We gather her husband is on the staff here."

Peter reached for the phone and waved his hand to the police to continue talking. "I'm just going to check to make sure she's in good hands." Joshua leaned forward in his seat. "We're certainly shocked, Captain, and deeply saddened. Do you have any ideas yet as to why or how it happened?"

Captain Wong shifted and rubbed the badge on his chest. His deep-set brown eyes locked in momentarily on his colleague's. They nodded. He turned his gaze to Joshua. "This is off the record, Dr. Caliban. If my boss ever got wind of it, I'd be dead. But you took special care of my mother when she was dying."

Joshua nodded and snapped his fingers as he made the connection. "I'm sorry. I was preoccupied when you introduced yourself."

"No worry. You see so many people, I'm sure, " he said. He reached into his pocket and removed two handheld dictaphones.

You'll both recognize these, I'm sure. You guys are forever dictating notes into them. These are somewhat special. They're ultra-sensitive, voice-activated recorders."

Peter squirmed. "You mean to say the whole fucking thing is on tape! That's the ultimate in kinkiness, the ultimate tool for blackmail."

"You've got that right, Dr. Albert. I haven't listened to them in great detail, but I've heard them enough times to have a pretty good idea what happened. It isn't a pretty picture and … it … seems to implicate you, Dr. Caliban. Your name is mentioned at several points."

Joshua stared right at the end of his rope. Could he turn that rope into a life preserver or would it continue to feel like a noose around his neck? He took a deep breath. "How, may I ask, am I implicated?"

Captain Wong set a recorder on the desk. "It's highly irregular, but if you have the time now, I can play the tapes for you. I can fast forward through the parts which just picked up the video porn in the background."

Joshua glanced perfunctorily at the clock on his desk again, then nodded. Captain Wong hesitated, his eyes darting once more in Peter's direction.

"It's all right, Captain Wong. Dr. Albert is my trusted colleague and … uh … he's treating me for the drug problem I suspect is suggested on the tape."

Joshua smiled at Peter. Peter sighed, nodded, and smiled back. "A time to heal" he mouthed.

The scene the captain had described sounded like Sesame Street compared to what Joshua and Peter heard for the next ten minutes. Elaine MacDonald's blood-curdling scream on the heels of her previously recorded phone message was Captain Wong's signal to his colleague to turn off the tape. Joshua was shocked beyond words.

Peter spoke first. "We're very grateful for you sharing the tape with us, Captain. We understand that you've done so completely off the record. Is there any way we can keep the press off our necks until the details of your investigation are confirmed?"

"Yeah, the last thing you guys need is anymore bad press. Listen, no one could've taken better care of my mother than you did, Dr. Caliban. I can buy us a couple of days with informing next of kin. Besides, until we get back our lab reports, I can't be certain if both deaths were accidental overdoses or what."

Joshua's intercom buzzed. "Yes, Mary. What is it?"

"The ICU called. Mrs. Caliban is waking up. I thought you'd want to know."

Joshua's heart was racing. "I'm on my way," he said, standing up. "You'll have to excuse me. My wife is just waking up from surgery." Joshua turned to Peter and stared at the floor. "Can you come with me, Peter?"

"No. There are a few details I'd like to go over with the detective and the captain. Besides, you two need some time alone. Just be sure to ask Mary for the prescription I ordered."

Joshua started out the door but suddenly stopped to face Captain Wong. Taking the captain's right hand in both of his own, Joshua stood silently for a second.

"I'm grateful for all you've done to help, Captain."

Captain Wong cleared his throat. "As am I, Dr. Caliban."

Joshua walked over to the pile of clothes crumbled behind his bathroom door. Stooping down, he removed a slightly damp unopened letter from his shirt pocket and stuffed it into his green trousers. As he walked to the door, he turned and winked at the captain.

"Be careful of this guy, Captain," Joshua said eyeing Peter as he spoke. "He was Detective Colombo in an earlier life." Turning to leave, he added, "I'll see you in the boardroom shortly, Colombo."

Twenty-Four

Ruth sensed Joshua's presence even before she opened her eyes, and it was wonderful to see his graying beard and silver hair above her. No one had hands as big as his, no one could make her feel so safe and secure. She felt great relief at waking up to find herself still alive, but it was dampened by the memory of the loneliness she'd felt a few hours ago. She remembered watching the first drips falling down the tubing of the IV into her veins, without feeling Joshua's presence wrapped around her. It was more painful to her than any invasion of the knife.

Neither of them could speak at first. The silence of the room was punctuated only by their breathing and the steady hum of the machines hooked to her body. Ruth squeezed Joshua's hands, the tears streaming down her face. Joshua blinked his eyes to squeeze out the tears welling up inside them.

"How much, Joshua? How much did Peter have to cut? This bandage is too massive to see anything under and I'm too numb to feel it, " Ruth said, looking down her chin at her chest.

"Peter said he only had to remove a lump, " Joshua said shyly.

She smiled warmly and Joshua squeezed her hand in response. "And?" Ruth asked.

"Ross has the lump under his microscope now. Peter was cautious, but he felt confident that it was a clean cut."

Except for Ruth's quiet sobbing as she continued to release her fears, they sat in silence again. So much still to discuss, but for now they basked in this small peace. Ruth released Joshua's hands. She tried to reach for a tissue to wipe her eyes, but unable to move her bandaged aching body, she motioned with her eyes for his help. He plucked one out of the box and handed it to her. The impish smile he loved so much and had come to take so much for granted emerged.

"So, I gather it's one of those 'time will tell' prognoses you guys are so famous for?"

Joshua grinned back. He leaned down to kiss her lips. With her free hand, Ruth tried to caress the back of his neck. Pain shot through her shoulder. "Not a good idea," she groaned.

Joshua took her raised hand in both of his and kissed her fingers. "I'm sorry, sweetheart. I'm terribly sorry for not being here this morning."

"I love you, Joshua, and I'll be able to forgive you … at some point. Peter cut out a piece of my breast and you, my heart. I'll never be whole again. Both will take a while to heal, " she said without anger.

Joshua's gaze shifted from Ruth's eyes to their locked hands. "I realized driving back this morning that I've never been all there for you. So many times … so many times I acted like I was listening and I was a million miles away. I'm not even sure I know how to."

Ruth looked up at Joshua. His narrowed eyes were open wider. The line etched into the middle of his forehead from countless frowns was less pronounced.

"What happened, Joshua? Tell me what happened. And … " Joshua held up his right hand like a witness being sworn in at a trial. The fierce look of pride that filled his eyes was tempered by a glint of humility. He reached into his shirt pocket with his left hand and pulled out a bottle of pills. The letter from Mrs. Wong fell unnoticed onto the edge of Ruth's bed.

"I know, I know. No half-truths. No missing pieces. In addition to these, " he said showing her the bottle, "my doctor, our doctor, has prescribed regular doses of rigorous honesty. "

Ruth studied the bottle. Joshua had taken the first step. He might stumble along the way, but he'd admitted he was powerless to go it alone. Joshua stroked his beard and began to recount to her the last twenty-four hours.

As Joshua's battle with the giant trout unfolded, Ruth's anger waned. His self-analysis reminded her of one of the reasons she'd fallen in love with him: When Joshua set his mind to it, he could do anything. He was a powerful man, so much so, that it seemed to frighten him. Ruth recognized that Joshua, like most people, was afraid of success almost as much as he feared failure. So as he spoke, she nodded in understanding and encouragement to keep him talking.

"Sweetheart, it sounds like you captured a trophy of great significance."

"I think so, Hon, but as you said, only time will tell." Joshua breathed deeply. "That's the easy part of the story."

Ruth's mind raced ahead. Was she about to hear Joshua hit his bottom? She gently dug her nails into the palms of Joshua's hands to encourage him to go on. "And what happened after that? What kept you from being here this morning?"

Joshua continued, his story generously sprinkled with sincere apologies, defensive rationalizations and excuses. "The damn watch broke when I fell. I should have thought to ask Peter to give me a wake-up call, just to be safe."

"I appreciate your honest apologies, Joshua. They're more important to me than I can tell you at the moment. But you consciously decided to get drunk and take the sleeping pills. What's important to me, to you, to us, to C.C.A. from now on are your actions, not your words."

Ruth watched as Joshua's normal angry, defensive reaction to her honesty rose to the surface. She watched expectantly as his Adam's apple flexed, and then relaxed.

"Fair enough, woman, " he said. "You get yourself healed and I'll show you some nonverbal action. And, stay tuned for the six o'clock news tonight. I guarantee it'll be better than the last one you taped."

Ruth forced a half-smile. C.C.A. hadn't been mentioned once yet. When was the last time Joshua had been so fully present? She could feel herself starting to fade out.

"I love you, Joshua, I love you so much. Give me a quick headline on what's happening with the suit and Damien before I doze off again."

"I love you, too, Ruth, more than I can tell you at the moment. I'm late for a vitally important board meeting. The headlines are that it's bloody. But I honest-to-God believe, though I can't even explain why, that everything is going to be okay. Can you trust that much until I can get back?"

Ruth's eyes were already closing. "Joshua, sweetheart. If I know you love me and are being honest with me, I can trust anything."

Joshua bent down and kissed her. "I'll try to get back after the board meeting, but it might be as late as half past six."

"Don't worry about me. Just give them hell and be dead honest. I'll be here when you get back."

As Ruth tried to adjust the pillow under her head, the letter from Mrs. Wong slipped to the floor. Joshua was moving too quickly to notice, and her eyes were already drooping. It would be there when Joshua got back.

❧

As he rushed out of Ruth's room, Joshua caught Allison Bridges, the floor nurse, looking at him. He had an unfamiliar urge to run over and hug her. A few weeks ago, Allison had been going to a wellness session. A hot, humid Saturday morning. Allison had gently chided Joshua and his colleagues for being too busy to attend to their own health. Joshua was rushing off to see Damien, sweater draped over his arm as protection against the weekend cold in the administration building, the same cold that contributed to Mr. LaPorte's pneumonia and ultimate death.

"Good morning, Allison. Sorry I didn't say hello before. I was anxious to see my wife."

"No sweat, Dr. Caliban. She seems to be doing fine. I'll be keeping a close eye on her."

Joshua had always been a leader who understood the value of being generous with praise for his workers, but this time there was more meaning than ever behind the words that came from his heart and not just his head. His legs felt wobbly again. He fumbled with his words as he shuffled toward Allison, arms outstretched. "I uh, I—just wanted to thank you for taking care of Ruth. It may be a few hours before I can get back to be with her."

Allison's jaw dropped and her blue eyes opened wide. "Don't worry, Dr. Caliban. We'll take good care of her." Allison added, blushing, "We're just doing our jobs."

Joshua lifted his hands from her shoulders and stuck them into his coat pockets. "Thank you, Allison. Thank you."

Joshua arrived at the boardroom fifteen minutes late, but he wasn't concerned. The delay would give everyone enough time to speculate on why the chairs normally occupied by Damien and Paul were empty. Given the grapevine at C.C.A., Lord knew what kind of rumors were racing around. For once, the rumors weren't likely to be anywhere near as dark and gruesome as the reality.

Joshua wanted desperately to take another of the withdrawal crutches Peter had given him, but the crushing intensity of the events exploding demanded his full attention, his total mental and emotional presence. Getting hooked on the pills made no sense. He'd have to handle the board meeting on his own two feet, wobbly as they were.

When he came into the room, he was struck by the sun gleaming off Moerae's golden blonde hair. Jane's flaming red hair next to her made the area to the right of Joshua's seat look like the blazing summer sun had settled at the head of the table. Mary rose to intercept Joshua before he sat down, to explain in a whispered message why Scott MacDonald's and Peter's seats were empty.

As everyone noticed Joshua's arrival, the animated buzzing rapidly dissipated. Judging from the somber looks and frowns, the grapevine had evidently been stretched to the limit. Joshua sat down and immediately leaned forward.

"There's no nice way to begin. C.C.A. is in a state of a code blue alert. Please bear with me, and I'll try to bring everyone up to date as quickly and clearly as I can. Let me start with Paul's and Damien's absence. They are both dead. Elaine MacDonald discovered their bodies."

Mary dropped her pencil into her lap.

"The details are sketchy but it appears that the cause of death is related to drug overdoses. The police will know more later. Scott is, I'm sure, trying to calm Elaine down. As you can appreciate, she's perhaps more shaken than the rest of us. Mary tells me that Peter has called to say he's tracking down some vital pieces of information. He'll join us as soon as he can." Joshua sat back. He'd had two hours to absorb the news. The rest of the board deserved a few minutes before he continued.

Jane broke the deathly silence. "The press is still breathing down our necks for some comment on the LaPorte suit. Are the police going to be able to keep this one away from them for a while?"

Ruth's words to be honest echoed in Joshua's mind. "We got lucky there," he said. "The police captain handling the case feels like he owes us one. We took care of his mother when she was dying a few weeks ago. He'll stall the press, at least for a while, so they can inform the next of kin."

"It might actually take some of the heat off the focus on the suit, " Jane said. "Besides, the likelihood of word not getting out is slim."

Joshua looked around the room. Everyone knew Jane was referring to the fact that Scott MacDonald had a mouth like a sieve. In this particular case, however, it was in Scott's best interest to keep his mouth shut. Joshua was counting on that.

"Can I leave this one for now?" Joshua said. "There are other crises pending that we may be able to do something about. "

Everyone nodded.

"The first has to do with getting the likes of Virgil Carter and Ashton Simons out of our hair."

"Getting leaches off your body would be easier, " Jane said. "What did you have in mind, Joshua?"

In five minutes he outlined his strategy for the power brokers. Roger Rosen curled his bottom lip over his penciled mustache. "That's a pretty dramatic ultimatum to lay in front of them, Joshua. If it backfires, we could go down in flames."

Moerae leaned forward and raised her eyebrows. "If I might, Dr. Rosen?" she said.

Joshua interrupted, "The kind of testimony someone like Moerae could be asked to provide would be an integral part of the trial. I've asked her to commit to working on our side. Please go ahead, Moerae."

"I'm convinced," Moerae began, "and I believe Jane concurs, that the only way to prevent C.C.A. from going down in flames is to follow the strategy Dr. Caliban has worked out. If we're right, the public is fed up with the prevailing win-lose business ethic. C.C.A. could become the leading edge of a whole new corporate attitude with implications that could potentially reach far beyond the health care industry."

Roger shook his bullet-shaped head hard and waved his hands. "If! If! And if we are wrong? I'd like to believe what you say, Moerae. But if we're wrong we'll be leading a stampede of helpless cattle being driven over the edge of a huge cliff." Roger's brow was beaded with perspiration in spite of the air conditioning blowing through the room.

Peter walked into the room.

"Yes, that's certainly possible, Roger," Joshua said. "This board, or what's left of it, may decide on a different strategy. What's critical to me," … Joshua paused. Was he really going to voice the words on the tip of his tongue? Had countless dreams and years of hard work come down to this one grain of truth? Joshua cleared his throat before continuing, "What's critical to me is that I'm convinced the charges against us are fundamentally true. If I'm to continue as C.C.A.'s president, any strategy we decide to implement must stem from that fact."

Roger Rosen's ebony eyes gazed unflinchingly at Joshua. Joshua shuddered. The last time he'd seen eyes like that was less than twenty-four hours ago, when Joshua was about to release the largest trout he'd ever dreamed of catching.

Roger leaned forward as he spoke. "How can we help, Joshua? What can we do to support you?"

Joshua looked away, rubbed his temples, and sighed. "Jane, Moerae, Peter, and I will have to meet after we're done. We need to prepare ourselves for the big boys' arrival. You, Ross, and Mary will need to figure out how to minimize the shock waves our people will feel when the word about Damien and Paul gets out.

"I'm going to ask Jane to call a news conference for five-thirty today. We'll touch base before then."

"It won't be a hard conference to organize, " Jane said, with a short laugh. "There's been a horde of them swarming around our front door all morning."

Still standing, Peter said, "I've got some important updates."

Joshua caught Peter's hazel eyes gazing at him. Peter's brows lifted imperceptibly looking for some clue as to what had transpired in the meeting thus far and how open he could be.

"I've filled everyone in on the police's verbal report about Damien and Paul. I'll fill you in on the LaPorte strategy afterwards. What have you got?"

Uncharacteristically, Peter started with the darkest news first. "After the police left, I immediately had Medical Records send me Damien's and Paul's complete histories. I was shocked to find an AIDS entry in Damien' s records."

"Jesus," Ross said. "He had AIDS?"

"It gets worse," Peter continued. "I got suspicious because, although the entry was dated months ago, the ink looked fresh. A friend of mine in police forensics was doing some more definitive tests, but early indications are that the entries were no more than a few days old."

"You mean they're phony?" Roger asked, "Why in God's name would anyone want to fake having AIDS?"

A sick wave washed through Joshua's gut. Peter proceeded to outline the scope of the insurance scam with Care, Inc. "When I saw the entry, I called the president of Care, Inc. The bottom line is that they would be, and I quote, 'more than happy' to make a donation to our nonprofit foundation to the tune of one million dollars, the exact amount they stand to receive as the prime beneficiaries of Damien's life insurance policy. In return, they expect us not to blow the whistle on them."

Joshua turned to Jane. "What's your instinct on this one, Jane? I realize, of course, you'll need to study the situation very carefully before you can render a formal opinion!"

"From a legal point of view, the business they're in is probably legit. The patients are getting what they asked for. Ethically, it sucks. But if we can help them relieve their guilt and do some good at the same time, I'd love to find a way. I'll look into it as soon as I can."

Joshua knew from experience that that meant they'd have an answer before the end of the day. "What else do we need to cover right now?"

Moerae looked at him expectantly. "These organizational matters are very important," she said, "but a dear friend has just come out of surgery. I don't think I'm alone in wanting to know how Ruth is."

"Her doctor tells me he's very pleased with the early results," Joshua said. "What's the final word, Ross?"

"I've checked and double-checked the lump Peter removed. As far as I can tell, he got it all, God willing."

Mary, who hardly ever spoke at normal board meetings without being spoken to, sighed with relief. "Lump? You did say lump, Dr. Benson?"

"I was able to leave over half the breast intact, " Peter said. We were very lucky." He smiled broadly. Looking over at Joshua, he added, "The Chief Bwana gave me explicit instructions in that regard."

A hearty laugh rolled round the table as everyone took a deep breath, especially Joshua. He cleared his throat conspicuously. The room fell silent. "I have one other question, Ross. Does … does … uh, the Impaired Physician's Committee still meet on Wednesday afternoons?"

Ross Benson's mouth dropped open. Then he nodded, his avocado eyes gazing warmly at Joshua. "Yes, we do, Joshua. Six p.m. every Wednesday. Tonight, in fact. Only now we call ourselves the Impaired Persons Committee. We've discovered that it's not only our physicians who are susceptible. We'd be honored to have you drop by and visit any time."

"I'd like to drop by this afternoon, if I may," Joshua said.

"We'll look forward to seeing you."

Joshua looked around the room at the friendly, warm faces. A scant hour-and-a-half from now, the air in the room wouldn't be filled with such love and understanding. He'd earned another of the pills Peter had given him.

"If there's nothing else on people's minds, we've all got a lot of work ahead of us," he said.

Joshua stood and the rest of them followed suit, forming a loose circle. Then Joshua extended his right hand to the center of the circle, and each one understood. They likewise put their right hands in, one on top of the other. No one spoke a word.

Twenty-Five

Joshua stared at the stuffed trout and nodded. The one he had released was almost twice its size. The plan Moerae had just outlined was simple. Joshua would arrive at the meeting late, using the excuse that he had to visit with Ruth. Even the hardest and coldest of hearts would understand that. Peter, Jane, and Moerae would arrive on time at four o'clock. They formed the advance unit invading enemy territory. Each of them was assigned a specific task to take individual guests aside and talk informally with them until Joshua arrived.

Joshua would drop the bombshell. In order for him to target the area where he'd have the greatest impact, the four had worked out an elaborate, covert signaling system to identify where the greatest resistance could be found.

Joshua had resisted Moerae's idea at first. Under enough pressure already, he was convinced that launching a four-pronged attack into a critical, highly sensitive meeting might result in his losing control and, ultimately, the meeting exploding in his face. But Peter and Jane both unequivocally sided with Moerae.

Moerae's persistence finally prevailed. "You hired me to be your corporate shrink and now you're resisting my advice," she said to him. He couldn't help but laugh and surrender graciously.

"This day will go down in C.C.A.'s history as Ultimatum Day," he said.

Jane had been assigned Shelly Jackson, chairperson of the Young Presidents Club, as she had helped Shelly win the election and write her acceptance speech. The first woman to hold the position, Shelly wielded enormous power in the business community.

The platform upon which she had run for election last year included a direct challenge to her CEO colleagues. "As long as there is a presumed distinction between business ethics and personal ethics, people will have every right to continue to mistrust the motives of America's corporate leaders." With great passion, she had further pleaded that the metaphoric language of Wall Street communicated a clear image of American industries' dominant values. "Corporate raiders," "hostile takeovers," "making a killing," and "head hunting" weren't the kind of ideas she believed the Young Presidents of Chicago should be supporting.

Joshua and his cohorts were confident of Shelly Jackson's support. She understood that the bottom line was the same in all organizations. Without people, organizations would not exist at all.

Peter persuaded them that misery loved company, so he'd take on Andrew Polanski and Ashton Simons together. They were sure to gravitate toward each other as soon as they arrived anyway. They'd have a lot to commiserate about. The lead article on the front page of USA TODAY stated that a probe of fifteen hospitals conducted by the Health and Human Services inspector general had uncovered over forty-two million dollars in unallowable Medicare charges.

The charges were accumulations of little things. A twelve hundred dollar charge for candy to lure doctors into a California hospital to prepare bills; a four-hundred dollar bill for supplying a Springfield, Illinois, physician's lounge with oranges to promote the idea of wellness.

Polanski and Simons, the commissioner of insurance and the president of Big Blue, respectively, would be crying on each other's shoulders. As third-party payers, they were about to get the third degree on the reimbursements they'd authorized when they came under the inspector general's careful scrutiny. Who knew what his audit might turn up?

Peter was confident he could handle the double duty of taking on both these men. "Between Ashton's girth and Andrew's self-esteem," he joked, "they probably won't even notice a shrimp like me." He had an ace up his sleeve provided by Hal Mays. Trumping any resistance the two insurance dealers might muster would give him great pleasure.

The last person to be assigned was Virgil Carter. He resembled a dull, gray, thick-skinned fish. Predators of the deep, sharks were known for their uncanny ability to sense when a man onboard ship was going to die. Rapacious and crafty, they followed the scent of blood for miles, waiting for the burial.

The conspirators thought that assigning Jane, a fellow shark, to Virgil would arouse his suspicion, especially since the two of them had yet to hold a civil conversation for longer than five consecutive minutes.

Moerae was thrilled at the opportunity to soften up Virgil. Joshua was afraid she'd be eaten alive, but Moerae could take care of herself. She argued that she had Greek blood in her veins, and the dolphin, the shark's only natural enemy, was a talisman from her Greek heritage. She wouldn't hesitate, she'd said with a flirtatious smile, to use feminine guile to out-charm the old snake charmer.

Joshua locked his fingers together and cracked his knuckles. The thought of Virgil Carter getting outfoxed brought a smirk to his lips.

Just before they broke to head for the showdown, Jane offered Moerae a last bit of advice. "Just remember, if the shark attacks, the best way to defend yourself is to smash him on the nose." Then she gave Moerae a clipping from the morning paper. "And if you really need to rub his nose in something, this might help." Jane smiled.

According to the article, the CEO of a major corporation had hung a huge, framed poster in the lobby of the corporate head-quarters. In bold print, the message read, "WARNING!! ATTORNEYS WILL BE SHOT. SURVIVORS WILL BE SHOT AGAIN."

Although the article gave them a good laugh, their mood was still sober. The erosion of the nation's spirit paralleled the plummeting fall from grace that both the legal and medical professions had suffered in recent decades. Lawyers were rapidly joining the ranks with physicians in the love-hate relationship between themselves and the public at large. Virgil Carter's personality was well suited to fanning the flames of mistrust, so Moerae's efforts would be critical to their ultimate success this afternoon. They all sincerely wished her luck.

Joshua looked up at the clock on the desk in his office. Another five minutes and he could head for the boardroom, too. He leaned back and smiled. When his three cohorts had left for the meeting, Joshua had half-heartedly lamented, "What am I going to do with myself for the next fifteen minutes? Twiddle my thumbs?"

Moerae had shoved the Bible she always carried in her bag into his hands. "Thumb through this. It will help to ground you.

The worn leather binding felt comforting even in his awkward grip. "Any sections in particular?"

Moerae just shrugged and lifted her neatly plucked eyebrows.

Joshua leafed through it until the two passages, in the Old Testament book of Joshua no less, caught his eye. Moerae had marked them with Post-It notes. Still skeptical, he nevertheless could trust Moerae's instincts. The messages might stand him in good stead in the battle ahead.

The nation of Israel was suffering for having fallen out of favor with the Lord. The reason? Achan, great grandson of Zerah of the tribe of Judah, had taken some gold and silver from the defeated warriors of Jericho. Not only had Achan done this against the Lord's explicit instructions, but he'd lied about it and hidden the loot among his own belongings.

Joshua's stomach tightened. Was it inevitable that an entire nation be punished for the sins of one man? Would all of C.C.A. as an organization suffer a similar fate because of his transgressions, just as the people of Israel did for Achan's?

What about his own 'tribe' of Hippocrates, the father of medicine? Would the entire medical profession be held accountable for the few bad apples in the barrel, for the few who stole gold and silver? Wasn't the tribe responsible for policing its own?

The second passage, toward the end of the book balanced the terrible sense of responsibility evoked by the first. He read that the Lord had accounted for the fact that His handymen were imperfect. He'd designated Cities of Refuge, where a man who accidentally killed someone could live and function among its inhabitants. As long as the man remained within the city's walls, he was guaranteed protection from the anger and revenge of the deceased's family. Should the high priest who was in office at the time of the accident die, the person was then free to return to his own home, the penalty having been paid.

Joshua's heart beat rapidly. How sad that the current malpractice mania left no room for such a refuge in modern times. Enormous resources were being drained away from direct patient care as a result. By some estimates he had read, thirty percent of the health care dollar was being spent on paperwork, and most of that was just covering someone's ass.

Defensive medicine was very expensive, and not only in dollar terms. Research had recently shown that medicine practiced in that way actually increased, rather than decreased, the probability of disease.

What kind of refuge could he and his colleagues seek from the inevitable, yet accidental losses that were bound to occur as they dealt with life and death every day?

Ought they be accountable for everything that took place within the walls of the organizations they headed? Would the meeting about to be held contribute toward establishing a cooperative way of life, rather than the adversarial one that affected every encounter today?

Joshua closed the Bible. Thousands of years ago, upon the death of Moses, another Joshua, the son of Nun, had been given the leadership of the nation of Israel. He had heard long ago that "Joshua" meant "God saves" in Hebrew. Recently, Moerae told him that the Greek equivalent in mythology meant "courage." He knew that he needed a healthy supply of both.

In the boardroom, the three meetings were well underway. With an imperceptible nod, Peter acknowledged Joshua's arrival. Ashton and Andrew kept on chattering. Joshua read Peter's other signals as confirmation that the insurance wheels would squeak and squeal but wouldn't buck the tide.

Facing the door, Jane made no attempt to hide the fact that she had seen Joshua come in. Her right hand moved to an imaginary hat, take it off and send it sailing through the air. Joshua returned her smile as he interpreted the gesture: The chairperson of the Young Presidents Club was likely to throw her hat enthusiastically into the ring with C.C.A.

A clean sweep was more than Joshua could have expected, so he wasn't really surprised by Moerae's covert message. She had a remarkable ability to appear blind to something right in front of her eyes. Even though she looked for all the world like Virgil

Carter had her full attention, she managed to convey both acknowledgment and ignorance of Joshua's arrival at the same time. By this she indicated that the president of the Bar Association could not only be counted on to hiss and rattle like a snake, but that his venomous strikes could be potentially inflict significant harm.

Ruth's last admonition to Joshua had been that he be dead honest. But being completely honest with Virgil Carter could be suicide. Under the guise of giving information, Joshua might really be intimidating; while seeming to consult, he would be applying coercion. Ruth would have to forgive him.

Joshua started speaking even before he sat down at the head of the table. "Thank you very much, ladies and gentleman, for joining us on such short notice. My apologies for being late. My wife had major surgery this morning. And ... " he paused as if trying to control his emotions, "to be perfectly frank, I spent the last few minutes reading the Bible."

The conspirators had rehearsed the possibility that Joshua might make such a seductive statement for his entry, or else they wouldn't be able to maintain straight faces at that last bit of frankness.

Ashton's face registered confusion and Andrew's and Shelly's flushed with what looked like genuine concern. So far, so good. Virgil's square jaw dropped at hearing Joshua's opening words. It was a look he didn't wear well. Just as he'd done so many times to witnesses on the stand, Virgil had allowed himself to be led down the garden path under Moerae's skillful manipulation. Having gleaned two pieces of information from Joshua that Ruth was very ill and Joshua had just read from the Bible, Virgil's mind jumped to a logical, but false, conclusion.

"Is she ... is she going to be all right?" Virgil's hand shot up to his lips and his normally furrowed brow flattened.

Joshua could barely suppress a smile. Virgil had a heart under that rough veneer after all. No harm in cultivating it a bit more.

"We certainly hope so, Virgil. Thanks for asking." Joshua turned his attention to the entire group. "Under the circumstances, you'll all forgive me, I know, for getting right to the point. At five-thirty this evening, C.C.A. has called a news conference to make its first public response to the charges involved in the LaPorte case, a case with which I know you are all familiar.

"As you can imagine, we have studied the situation very thoroughly. The case could set an entirely new precedent that would effect us all deeply. Under these circumstances, we're hoping to avail ourselves of your counsel on the general parameters of our position. Totally off the record, of course."

Andrew Polanski removed his glasses, breathed on them, and wiped them clean with his tie. Did he realize the scope of the impact that the case could have on his industry? A domino effect would immobilize first the insurance carriers and then the providers themselves. The courts would be choked with suits, putting the entire system in gridlock.

Andrew and Ashton wouldn't be the only ones to fear this sequence of events either. Win or lose, the case would certainly put a giant hole in C.C.A.'s financial underbelly. Should the jury ultimately rule against C.C.A., a precedent would be set that could engender a torrent of related cases, wreaking havoc on the entire health industry.

Andrew's interests were at stake here, too. He'd put aside any ambivalent feelings he might harbor toward Joshua and help him beat this challenge. "We certainly hope you're successful in settling this ludicrous case out of court, Joshua," he said. "There would never be enough in our reserves to cover the flood of claims such a negative ruling could unleash. We'd all have the government in our hair even more than we do now."

Joshua couldn't believe their luck. The meeting had hardly begun and Andrew had already made himself vulnerable to the bomb Hal Mays had prepared for Peter. At Peter's request, Hal had done some arms-length computer modem research. From the comfort of his home, Hal had easily gotten into the financial records of all the third-party payers who served Chicago.

Playing the float was not unique to Big Blue. All the major third-party payers seemed to have their own unique ways of maximizing premium income while minimizing the speed of reimbursements. The commissioner of insurance would be aware of how common these shady practices were. If Hal's findings were any indication, the commissioner was in on a few deals himself.

"Come, come," Peter said to Ashton and Andrew, as if he were mildly chastising two teenagers for coming home an hour late. "You guys don't expect any sympathy from us on your profit reserves, do you? Everyone knows that the real profit you make is in the float from tardy reimbursements to providers and policyholders. Government auditors would have no trouble documenting that fact, particularly if they also had subpoenas for provider reimbursement applications."

Joshua watched Ashton intently as Peter let that little jab sit and fester before putting on his most innocuous Colombo demeanor and delivering the final blow.

Peter's hazel eyes locked in on Ashton. "What was it last year, Ashton? Something like 4.275 million, wasn't it?"

If Peter had said several million, Ashton could have passed it off as a good guess. Accusations were one thing, but correct figures to the third decimal point were quite another.

"Damien should never ..." Ashton said before he could catch himself, his mouth gaping in shock.

Andrew Polanski bit his lower lip and shook his head hard. Joshua glanced at Peter and nodded slightly. Peter's bomb had made a direct hit. Some kicking and screaming was to be expected, but they were assured of support from the insurance boys now.

"'Peter the Rabbit,' we call him," Joshua said, smoothing feathers adroitly. Peter had really detonated a land mine. "He's always pulling numbers out of his hat. The key point is that you two and the insurance industry in general have as much at stake in this case as C.C.A."

Thank God Captain Wong had made good on his word. No one had even intimated they'd heard anything about the police investigation, so he was assured that the details of the deaths of Damien and Paul had not leaked out yet. Their strategy dictated that he and his allies exert pressure in this meeting before the news conference took place, but Joshua wanted to avoid overt warfare.

Shelly Jackson leaned forward, resting her elbow on the table and chin in her hand. "Joshua, I hate to show my ignorance, but I, for one, know very little about the case to which you've been referring. All I know is what I heard on the news the other night and, of course, the scuttlebutt passed around La Bonheme. I'd like to be supportive, but I don't know how to help."

"Oh, I apologize," Jane said, before Joshua could respond. "I was supposed to fill you in before the meeting." Turning to the rest of the group, Jane continued, "I got totally absorbed in Shelly's story from Charles Sykes' book, A Nation of Victims. It's actually quite germane to our agenda. Would you mind repeating it, Shelly?"

Shelly sat erect and straightened her Cleopatra-cut blond hair. "Well, you all know what a buzzword 'codependency' has become these days. Sykes tells a story about a guy who lost his job because he could never get to work on time. The attorney argued that his client was handicapped by chronic lateness syndrome, which was rooted in his dysfunctional family. The attorney argued and won his client's reinstatement! Complete with full back pay and damages!"

"Unless you're just setting up for another round of the new American pastime, lawyer bashing, I must say I miss the point of that story, Shelly," Virgil said, not even trying to mask his flippancy. He didn't even wait for a response. "In fact, Joshua, I'm at a loss as to why you've even asked us here. You've already got a house full of attorneys whose future livelihood depends on winning the LaPorte case. Are you fishing for some really expert advice for free? In my fraternity, we call that 'judicial liposuction'."

Joshua ignored the sting Virgil's arrogant barb, and swallowed a volley of cutting rejoinders. Jane was smiling and biting her lip. Revenge would be that much sweeter for the waiting.

Joshua had sworn that he'd rather see C.C.A. go down in flames than ask someone like Virgil Carter for help, but he needed him. As much as he hated to admit it, Joshua knew the strategy he and the board had agreed to take required Virgil Carter's acquiescence. Without it, C.C.A. might go down anyway.

"Feel free to bill me for your time if you must, Virgil." Joshua looked away from Virgil and spoke again to the group. "I'm asking for feedback on the strategy we've committed ourselves to follow in regards to the LaPorte case. All of the options we've identified have implications that influence all of you."

"I'd be happy to give you the benefit of my experience, pro bono if need be," Virgil said with a crafty smile. "But do you really think these busy people need to hear all the legal details of your defense? Not that beating down an accusation of managerial malpractice should be all that hard."

In a measured and unwavering tone Joshua stated, "At five thirty today, C.C.A. is fully prepared to announce its culpability in this case—'guilty as charged'!"

Ashton Simons nearly jumped out of his seat. "That's insanity!"

Virgil Carter bolted up at the same instant. "You can't be serious, Joshua?"

"I'm dead serious."

Virgil wrung his hands nervously and looked up and down the table several times, shaking his head. "Why would you plead guilty? Why would you throw in the towel without a fight?"

Joshua repressed a snide reply. He swallowed hard so as not to allow his dislike of Virgil to cloud the air. His team had agreed before the meeting that Jane, Peter or Moerae would play the role of the hard guy with Virgil rather than himself. A standard negotiating ploy designed to knock the opponent off guard.

Joshua didn't want to lie outright. Neither could he kowtow to a man he distrusted. Let he who is without sin cast the first stone. Joshua let go a little more.

"You're right, Virgil," he began. "There was a time when throwing in the towel would never have entered my mind. People and circumstances have convinced me that the insanity to which you referred, Ashton is industry-wide. Indeed, it's nation-wide. It must stop. The simple answer to your question, Virgil, is that C.C.A. is guilty of the charges being brought by the LaPorte family. Through acts of commission and omission, we at C.C.A. have behaved in uncaring ways toward each other and our patients. Beginning with myself and my colleagues on the board, we haven't been treating each other as well as we know how."

No one had ever seen Virgil at a loss for words, but then Joshua had never before told Virgil he was right. He backed down glaringly into his seat. He looked like a trial lawyer stunned by a judge's warning that any further objections would be overruled.

Ashton leveled a finger at Joshua. "It was your state of sanity I was questioning, Joshua! Not the industry's!"

Joshua glanced at Moerae. She'd been observing carefully, waiting to find an appropriate time to enter the battle. If Virgil had followed his M.O. during their tête-à-tête before the meeting started, he'd have put the make on her in ten minutes.

The time was ripe for her to cash in some of those chips. "May I?" Moerae asked, looking at Ashton as if she were seeking his permission. Ashton may not have cared to be stroked by Joshua, but attention from Moerae was something else.

A huge smile appeared on his round red face. "Please, Dr. King. Maybe you can talk some sense into his head."

"Actually, Mr. Simons, I was personally pleased to hear you use the word insanity. Dr. Caliban reacted defensively the first time I used the same term. We'd been talking about the state of human affairs in most organizations."

Moerae paused and glanced at Joshua. She thought she caught a hint of a grin. Virgil folded his hands. He was a tough man in his own estimation, but he loved women who could be tough with men. He was listening carefully.

Moerae stood up. "Can you give me a better definition of 'insanity' than the conscious repetition of behavior known to bring destruction and failure? Workaholism is as potentially lethal an addiction as any we know. Dishonesty, equally so. Covering up mistakes, saying and doing things primarily because they please the boss, are common practices in organizations all over the nation.

"The automobile industry denied the threat of competition from the Japanese, and found themselves effectively shut out of their own domestic market. In the same way, patients deny their diseases. When an individual can't get past initial denial and lives in an irrational state of unreality, we call it insanity. When an organization acts that way, we simply rationalize it by calling it politics."

Shelly Jackson nodded. Ashton, Andrew, and Virgil were mesmerized. Moerae held the room captive. "Organizations don't do anything. People do. Don't you see? An organization can behave in an insane manner! Organizations are people!"

Moerae had made her points with Shelly, Andrew, and even Ashton. She still had to draw Virgil back into the conversation so that Joshua could deliver his final ultimatum. What would Virgil's reaction be? She engaged him with her eyes and extended a hand to him.

"You and I were agreeing on a related point before the meeting started," she began, "Remember? We both agreed with the bumper sticker: 'Guns don't kill people—people kill people."

Virgil suddenly grimaced and his face reddened. Joshua tensed up. Damn! Please don't let him recognize their ploy to use him as a pawn.

Virgil stood up and gathered his pad and pencil, poised and ready to move toward the door. "I agree with Andrew. This whole meeting is insane. If you're serious, Joshua, it will set a precedent that will destroy the health care industry as we know it. I, for one, think it's time to leave."

"The insurance industry would become nonexistent!" Andrew moaned.

"You're going to commit suicide and take the rest of us down with you." Ashton nodded.

Shelly Jackson, on the other hand, was radiating hope and enthusiasm. "I couldn't disagree more, Andrew," she said. "I believe the implications of what Joshua is driving at could breathe new life into the business world overnight! Imagine, the way we treat people being as important as the bottom line! Did I hear you right, Joshua; that you said C.C.A. was fully prepared to admit its guilt?"

Joshua let the momentary silence hang as Virgil stared at him. "We're prepared to admit our guilt," Joshua repeated, "because we are guilty. Under management's direction, C.C.A. has ignored its own wellness, its own health, as a human organization. As a business in the business of providing humane health, we allowed ourselves to neglect ourselves. We are further convinced that the entire health care industry, indeed, industry at large, is suffering from the same illness."

Joshua paused to take a drink of water. His throat felt very dry. The last time it had felt this dry had been last evening. Then, he had soothed his thirst with a half bottle of bourbon.

"You know," he continued in a warmer tone, "there's an old Hippocratic aphorism I've never forgotten: 'Wherever the art of medicine is respected, there is also respect for humanity.' It seems to me that the reverse is true for life in general: Wherever there is respect for the sacred nature of humanity, there is also respect for the art of any endeavor, of any industry."

Joshua turned directly to Virgil Carter. He gazed expectantly into his steeled eyes. He slowly and deliberately turned his intent look to Ashton, and then to Andrew. He softened his expression as he turned to Shelly Jackson and his colleagues, but turned up the intensity when he returned to Virgil Carter. "Whatever our differences, I think we could agree that the public's respect for our respective professions is at an all time low. Doctor bashing has become as popular as lawyer-bashing, Virgil.

"I submit to you that the reason is that both professions have lost sight of the real bottom line, the only bottom line that really matters: respect for our humanity. If that's our society's illness, and we believe it is, then we have an opportunity to help heal the nation. We've sworn an oath. We have the responsibility to heal ourselves first."

Joshua paused to rub his eyes, leaving no doubt, even to Virgil, that he was sincere.

"I love this organization," he continued. "I love it like a father loves his son. I have done things in the past, both accidentally and with full awareness, to hurt it. If … if … it must die so that others can live a healthier life, then so be it."

Joshua turned to Jane. He was exhausted and didn't have the energy to go any further. He gestured for her to take over. Jane leaned a little in his direction, as if she were about to give him a hug, but stopped. She glanced up at the clock on the wall.

"Please bear with me," she began, "Our time is running very short. The four of you," she met each one's eyes before moving to the next, "have enormous power. Together, you could influence the shape of health care policies for the people of Chicago and even beyond.

"Mr. LaPorte's death was untimely, unfortunate, and sadly, avoidable. The family has no desire for vengeance, but they do deserve and expect to be compensated for their loss. The LaPortes are willing to settle out of court. Their proposal is straightforward." Jane paused.

"We must be prepared to announce that we've agreed to join forces to do everything humanly possible to ensure that Mr. LaPorte's death wasn't in vain," she continued. "We must tell the public that an unprecedented, collaborative effort will be initiated to ensure we learn from this tragedy. We must promise the people of Chicago that Mr. LaPorte's death will herald a new era in the humane quality of patient care."

Joshua scanned the eyes of the others in the room. Ashton and Andrew didn't like what they were hearing, but were resigned to the fact since a jury's verdict could bring much worse.

Shelly Jackson's smile covered her normally sphinx-like face. Virgil coiled, snakelike, and backed into a corner. He hadn't yet exhausted his venom.

"Well, that's certainly a dramatic proposal," he sneered. "You'll excuse the lawyer in me, but what exactly is involved in 'heralding in a new era and compensating the LaPortes for their loss'?"

"I can speak to the compensation issue," Jane responded.

"We're hoping that the final settlement is an amount we can cover together without having to draw from our formal insurance coverage. I'll let Dr. King answer your second question."

"Why, that's blackmail! " Andrew yelled.

"You can't get away with that! " Ashton seconded.

Peter leaned forward eagerly, and Ashton's portly face blanched. Andrew stiffened. Joshua had earlier received a check from Ashton covering all the late reimbursements stretching back for years, a virtual admission of guilt from Big Blue.

"Ashton, we'd like to thank you for your prompt balancing of our shortfall account. The interest due C.C.A. on those monies will be deferred to the LaPorte fund as part of your contribution, " Peter said smoothly.

Moerae jumped in: "On the question of improving the quality of care, C.C.A. has hired me to work with their people from the CEO at the top to the people at the bottom of the line. We intend to create an organizational culture that is totally and singularly focused on healing and caring. Dr. Caliban and his board have authorized me to work with a designated representative from each of your organizations to accomplish the same thing. We will share all of our successes and failures at C.C.A. and distribute our final report for you to use in transforming your own institutions."

"Freely! Pro bono, I might add!" Joshua said, smiling.

Virgil cleared his throat, loosened the knot on his tie, and shook a finger in the air. "I don't feel comfortable committing my practice without consulting them first," he said.

Moerae sat erect. But before she could open her mouth, Shelly Jackson surprised everyone by saying, "I suggest, then, that we tell the press who in turn will tell the people of Chicago that the legal establishment isn't on board, that it has taken our proposal under advisement," she said.

Ashton and Andrew slumped in their chairs. Virgil shot Joshua an appraising look, threw up his hands, and sat down. Joshua sighed. The last of the resistance had drained away.

The phone rang. Peter grabbed it. "Yes. Oh, hi, Mary. Of course. Right away." Peter hung up the phone and said to Joshua, "That was your office. Mrs. Caliban has awakened."

"Thank you, Peter. And I want to personally thank each and every one of you for your gracious willingness to join us." As he spoke, he looked each of them in the eye. "Jane and Peter will be representing C.C.A. at the news conference. You have only a few moments to work out the final wording of the announcement."

Joshua looked intently at Virgil Carter. "I do hope you'll Join with us, Virgil," he said sincerely. "There cannot be a more important issue of human justice than ensuring that every human being, patient or otherwise, is treated with the utmost care and respect. If you'll excuse me now, I must go."

Joshua got up to leave but stopped, silently looking around the boardroom. He'd been to more meetings in this room than he could count. The snapshots of C.C.A.'s history looked brighter today. His face reflected in the glass covering his own picture was more serene. Even the fish in the tank seemed to be swimming more freely. A warm feeling covered his heart as he took in the collage of hard-earned degrees of all C.C.A.'s doctors.

So few bad apples in the barrel.

Twenty-Six

Joshua was so preoccupied with his own thoughts, he never saw Kathy Marshall stepping out of the Nurses' Lounge. "Hey, we've got enough trouble without our own people suing us for injury," he said with a big smile as he stumbled to get out of Kathy's way.

"Oh, Dr. Caliban. I was just thinking of … oh, I'm sorry."

"No need to call your insurance company. I'm just headed to a meeting. What are you still doing around here?"

"I'm on a committee that meets Wednesday nights."

They both looked at each other, then quickly looked away.

"I have a hunch we might be headed for the same meeting," he said.

Kathy threw her arms around Joshua and hugged him. Joshua stared hard at his shoe tips. Kathy withdrew immediately, as discreetly as she could. She quickly dropped her arms and stiffened into a more formal posture. "Yes, I guess maybe we are, Dr. Caliban. We can walk separately if you'd like."

Joshua thought for a second, then reached out and hugged her back. "No, I don't think so, " he said, grabbing her elbow. "You saved two lives yesterday. One was mine. Let's go."

Kathy waved her hands as if to say it was no big deal. "As soon as I saw the thermo strips heating up, I knew something was wrong. How's Mrs. Caliban?"

"Thanks to the likes of you and Peter, it seems as though she's going to be fine. I'm headed back up to see her after our meeting."

"I'm glad to hear that, Dr. Caliban. We get a lot of help, however," she said, nodding toward the heavens. "We're only the technicians. He does the heavy work."

Joshua nodded as they entered the meeting room. Ross Benson and Anita Riccardo greeted him with warm smiles. Joshua had prepared himself for a large group including some people he might not have recognized. He was taken aback.

"Are we early?" he asked.

"No, no, Joshua. Anita, Kathy, and I are all you'll see this evening. We're part of a special subcommittee of the whole. Have a seat and I'll explain, " Dr. Riccardo said.

For the next five minutes they described how the committee functioned. Anita stressed that since preserving anonymity was essential, particularly for the doctors, they had formed this subcommittee. They were empowered to meet first with any impaired physician who wanted to talk.

"In most cases, " Ross interjected, "our subgroup is able to provide all the support that' s needed."

Joshua listened quietly to their briefing. He'd known about the committee, but knew little of the scope and magnitude of their contribution. Ross asked the first of the series of hard questions that followed.

"By the time a person gets to our committee, Joshua, the situation is pretty clear to everyone. For reasons we're sure you can appreciate, however, we need to hear in your own words why you've asked to speak with us."

Kathy, Ross, and Anita sat in respectful silence. In the poster hanging on the wall, a polio-stricken child had one hand on his walking stool. The other hand was reaching for the outstretched hand of a smiling parent, but the gap between them was too wide. The child would have to risk letting go to get where he wanted so badly to be. Joshua, too, would have to make that choice, to let go, alone.

Joshua ran through a myriad of rationalizations and excuses in his mind. A dysfunctional childhood, the stress of his job, Ruth's illness. Each of them presented a partial truth. But he knew in his heart that none of them was the whole truth. Joshua had faced an audience of thousands of strangers before and it never fazed him. Now, seeing the three familiar faces in front of him, all friends, he felt his knees shaking.

"I.. .uh...have.. .a problem. I think … ur … with drugs and alcohol."

Anita Riccardo, likely the next head of the anesthesiology department, leaned forward to speak. The contrast between Anita and Paul was dramatic, for she was as warm as he had been cold.

"Joshua, we want you to know that we appreciate how extraordinarily difficult and courageous it is for anyone to voluntarily come before this committee," she began. "I know I speak for my colleagues as well. We are honored that you would trust us enough to take this step. Hard as it may be for you to believe at the moment, I can assure you that the worst is probably over. To help us all know what the next steps ought to be, we need to ask you some additional questions."

The genuine empathy in Anita's voice made Joshua's mind ring. He could hardly believe the words he himself had just spoken and was confused not to hear a stream of punishing threats and accusations in reaction to his statement. All he could do was nod.

"When was the last time you had a mind-altering substance?" Kathy asked.

"You mean one I didn't prescribe for myself?" They all laughed. "Peter is managing my withdrawal and has prescribed accordingly."

They nodded.

"Joshua, are you aware of any effects on your ability to care for patients?" Ross sounded like a concerned friend rather than an inquisitor.

Joshua looked down at the table. He could answer the question, but he couldn't do so looking his colleagues in the eye.

"Were it not for Kathy Marshall, I might have lost a patient yesterday. I'm not sure it matters, but I don't think it was ever that bad before. Believe me, there's no way in hell I'll let it get that bad again."

Anita Riccardo sat up sharply. "Joshua, there are several prescriptive therapies we can offer." She outlined the most typical and told Joshua he would have to think them over and discuss them with his wife and with Peter. "You have to decide which one is best for you. All of them require total abstinence," she stressed, "and you must be relieved of your patient responsibilities for a period of time."

"I guess I was expecting that I'd be barred from my operating privileges for a while," Joshua said. Would his position as C.C.A. 's president have saved him from that fate? His tone took on a hint of exhaustion, resignation. "I plan to take the rest of the week off. When do you need my decision?"

Ross looked expectantly at his two colleagues. "Under the circumstances, would it be acceptable to the two of you if Dr. Caliban committed to informing me personally of his decision? By Monday morning? I'd fill you both in myself."

Kathy and Anita looked at each other. Kathy spoke. "Perfectly okay. We'll leave him in your capable hands." Then she said to Joshua, "Please don't hesitate to contact either one of us if you want more details, Dr. Caliban."

"Dr. Caliban, you've just made a giant step forward toward healing, " Anita said. "If there's nothing else on the agenda tonight, Ross, I suggest we call it a day."

"I'm off to see my wife," Joshua said as he stood up. He laughed out loud before finishing his thought. "Otherwise, I'd offer to buy everyone a drink."

"Mind if I walk over with you?" Ross asked. "I won't stay long. Just want to bring you up to date on some things and say a quick hello to Ruth."

Joshua felt an uneasiness he couldn't identify. Maybe, like Ruth said, lying got in the way of loving people. A man couldn't be grateful if his spontaneity was curtailed by having to guard against half-truths all the time. Joshua grabbed Ross' hand in both of his. "We've walked through a lot together, my friend. I'd love the company … probably more than the update."

Nevertheless, as they walked toward Ruth's room, Ross summarized what had happened since their luncheon meeting. Captain Wong had promised to fill them in before he released any details to the press. Mary and Moerae meanwhile wrote up a series of internal announcements from which they could choose as soon as they heard from the police.

"What kind of announcements?" Joshua asked, frowning.

"We were a bit anxious about letting the cat out of the bag, " Ross said, "but Moerae convinced us to organize a program to facilitate a grieving process for our employees. She helped us see that no matter how we may feel toward Paul and Damien, they were human beings who gave a lot of themselves to C.C.A."

"It sounds like a good idea, I guess," Joshua didn't sound totally convinced. "What does Moerae recommend?"

"She offered to personally conduct small group meetings to help people let go of whatever feelings might have been triggered by the two deaths. I think her idea is super. It'll help control the rumor mill, which may already be gearing up. No doubt it'll be working overtime once the news breaks."

"I agree," Joshua said. He abruptly stopped. A patient in a nearby room was tuned in to the six o'clock news. Joshua had picked up Virgil Carter's unmistakable, familiar voice on the tail end of the C.C.A. story: "… and we're in total agreement that there can be no more important issue of human justice than ensuring that every human being, patient or otherwise, is treated with the utmost care and respect."

Next they heard the voice of Carol Russell, the station's anchorwoman. "Well, there you have it, ladies and gentlemen. We, and all the people of Chicago are simply stunned. It is an unprecedented and very dramatic move. Representatives of the legal profession, the insurance industry, and the business community at large have joined with C.C.A. in an effort to use the circumstances surrounding the death of famous restaurateur Mr. J.P. LaPorte to, and I quote, 'herald in a new era in the humane quality of patient care.'

"Garth Haskins, attorney for the LaPorte family, refused to release any details of the settlement to the press. Stay tuned for more reactions to today's dramatic news after a word from our sponsor."

"I can't believe that was Virgil Carter talking," Ross said as they started off down the hall again. "What in the hell did you guys do to him this afternoon?"

Joshua shrugged. His own words had most definitely emerged on national TV from Virgil Carter's mouth. "Lord knows, but it sounds like the rest of the news is just as sweet," Joshua said, nodding toward the party-like noise emanating from Ruth's room.

Joshua and Ross found Ruth watching the weather report, propped up in her bed. She was looking remarkably bright and cheery. Mary, Jane, Moerae, and Peter were all squeezed together, craning their necks to get a good view of the TV screen.

"Doesn't anyone remember the policy on the number of visitors allowed in a room at one time?" Joshua asked as he leaned down to kiss Ruth. "It looks like Super Bowl party in here!"

Ruth blinked a tear from her burnt sienna eyes. Her arms entangled by IV tubing and monitor wires kept her from reaching up to grab him. He leaned down again and she planted a long, lingering kiss on his lips. Joshua's face was flushed as he stood up again.

"I invited some friends to a news-watching party!" she began, an indulgent smile warming her face. "Besides, I'm in pretty tight with the boss of this place. We taped it for you, Joshua. It was wonderful."

"Ross and I caught Virgil's closing remarks on the way over," Joshua said. "I could hardly believe my ears. What in God's name did you do to him before the meeting, Moerae?"

Moerae squirmed on the edge of the bed. An impish, little girl smile came over her face. "To tell you the truth, Joshua, I'm not sure. He tried to put the make on me right away as you predicted."

"Oh, tell us how," Mary interrupted with a gleeful smile. "I love a good soap opera."

"Nothing very creative. He tried the old 'are you a natural blonde' line."

Joshua grinned as he remembered wondering the same thing when he first laid eyes on Moerae. "And you said?"

"I gave him the standard response. 'Only my hairdresser, and lover, know for sure.' To which he responded, 'Why don't we get together for a drink sometime? I've been thinking about changing my career.'"

Everyone burst out laughing. The phone next to Ruth's bed rang. Peter grabbed it first. Covering the mouthpiece, he whispered, "It's Captain Wong. I gave him this number."

Joshua waved Peter to go ahead. An air of anxious anticipation settled heavily in the room. Everyone listened intently.

"Yes, we just watched it. Quite positive! No, we certainly don't want you to do anything against the law. That would be very kind and generous of you. Would you like to tell him yourself? I'm sure he will. Thank you, too, Captain."

As he hung up the phone, Peter's right thumb popped up and he winked at Joshua. "The coroner's report confirmed that Paul's death was from natural causes."

Ruth gasped, prompting Joshua to remember he hadn't yet told her the gory details. "You ... you'd just awakened from the operation a few minutes after I heard about it, Hon," he told her. He quickly filled her in on the circumstances of the gruesome deaths. When he was finished, he turned back to Peter.

"What did the captain say about Damien?"

"Damien clearly died of an overdose. But even after reviewing the tapes thoroughly, they can't be certain whether it was at Paul's hand or Damien's. Damien's prints were on the syringe but Paul had been wearing gloves and he could have put the syringe into Damien's hand."

Ruth frowned again at the mention of the tapes, so Joshua explained superficially what Paul had been up to. He watched the confusion on her face turn to chagrin but, anxious to let Peter finish, he only skimmed the story, hoping she'd understand he'd tell her more later.

"What was it the captain wanted to tell me himself, Peter?"

"That's why I made a thumbs-up! The captain doubts they'll ever be able to be sure about who caused Damien's death but, for now, he stressed that you and C.C.A. don't have to worry about being dragged in."

Joshua heaved a deep sigh and quietly reached down to grasp Ruth's open hand. How could he have been so lucky? "Where does that leave Elaine MacDonald?" Jane asked, putting two and two together.

"I saw Dr. MacDonald leaving the hospital with her just before I came up," Mary interjected.

"He was fuming. And if you'll pardon my cattiness, that was the first time I've ever seen them together when Elaine was the one on the tether-end of the leash and not her Scottie!"

Gales of laughter filled the room again.

"Speaking of people at the end of their rope, that reminds me," Jane said when the noise died down, "I followed up with Care, Inc. as Peter requested. They have graciously agreed to make a donation of one million dollars to the C.C.A. Foundation. They asked me what we're going to do with it. I told them you'd get back to them."

Ross let out a long, shrill whistle. "We shouldn't have any trouble figuring out what to do with a million bucks. On the other hand," he laughed, nodding in Joshua's direction, "the board will probably never be able to agree and it will end up back in the president's lap."

Ross's comment reminded all of them that the composition of C.C.A.'s board had changed quite dramatically in the past twenty-four hours.

Joshua nestled in closer to Ruth's side. The letter from Mrs. Wong sitting unopened on the floor beside Ruth's bed caught his eye. Still furious with Damien for getting the Wong family caught up in his greedy machinations, Joshua felt a sudden sadness for Damien that he didn't understand.

"I have a specific proposal I'll be trying to sell to the powers that be," he said. "I'm going to suggest that the C.C.A. Foundation support the Ruth J. Caliban Clinic in the creation of a therapeutic healing center for AIDS patients and their families." Ruth and Joshua squeezed each other's hands. "And since I'm in pretty tight with the boss of that place, I'm hopeful that I can talk her into it being called the Father Damien Room."

Ruth muted the TV set. The room suddenly fell very quiet. She looked at Joshua with tears in her eyes. Joshua bit his lip to stem the tears welling up in his. The idea had come to him while driving back from the cabin. He would take monies that had been garnered from the depth of a man's greed and avarice and would use them to offer comfort and spiritual healing for the terminally ill. A place of healing would replace Damien Rees' den of iniquity.

Few would know of the Damien Rees connection. Instead, the center's famous namesake would be Father Damien, the Belgian priest who had martyred himself in the Hawaiian Islands by selflessly serving a colony of lepers until he himself finally contracted and succumbed to the disease. Joshua and Ruth had both admired Father Damien as a symbol of compassion and service for many years.

Ross broke the silence. "I'm sure I speak for Peter and Jane as well as our new, yet-to-be named board colleagues. You will have our complete support."

Joshua had once felt sorry for himself because his job as CEO left him so little time to be a practicing physician, caring for patients. The events of the past few days had changed his thinking dramatically. He now realized that in his role as CEO, he had the opportunity to make an enormous impact on the quality of patient care that he would not have had in individual practice. C.C.A. was his patient, and he was its attending physician.

Ever since Ross had asked him if he was aware of any effects his addiction might have had on his ability to care for patients, Joshua knew what he had to do. He must excuse himself from his operating privileges in the boardroom as well as in the O.R. until he healed himself.

"For reasons you all know, and probably knew long before I admitted them to myself, Ross and his Impaired Persons Committee have recommended I take a break from surgery for awhile. I intend to follow their advice. In addition, effective immediately, I'm requesting the board to relieve me of my responsibilities as president. I will recommend that they name ...," he paused for a second to catch Peter's gaze, "... the little guy with brass balls as my successor."

Peter leaned back against Ruth's headboard. He locked the fingers of his hands together and cracked all of his knuckles, a big grin on his baby face. "Like I said to you once before, it's a big jockstrap to fill."

"If you'll pardon the pun, Peter," Jane said, leaning over to plant a kiss on Peter's forehead, "I want to echo what Ross just said. You'll have our complete support."

"If laughter is indeed healing, I believe Ruth will be discharged quite soon," Moerae said, wiping the tears from her eyes.

"Seriously, thank you," Peter said when they'd quieted down again. "I am honored and will need all the support I can get. The power brokers' meeting and the six o'clock news committed us to some gigantic challenges."

Ruth fidgeted slightly. "It's been a hell of a month today. All this excitement is getting to me. I'm only sorry I couldn't have been a fly on the wall at your meeting with the big boys. It sounds like it was magical. But right now, if you'll excuse me, I'd like to spend a little time with Joshua before taking a nap."

Peter stood up. "Joshua was magnificent. And just to make sure we were successful, I took out an insurance policy." He dropped his voice-activated tape recorder on the bed, winking at Joshua.

"Let me know how the instant replay sounded, then you can erase it!"

"Erase it, hell! It will be great research data for my next literary opus," Moerae said, rising from the end of the bed.

"You can take the woman out of academia, but you can't take academia out of the woman," Joshua said with a warm smile.

"It's your own fault, Joshua," Moerae said. "You authorized me to share all of our successes and failures."

"Pro bono," Jane added, as she, too, stood up next to Moerae.

"I don't know about sharing my personal battles with the whole world, though," Joshua began.

Moerae smiled. "Joshua, you're not unique in your struggles. We each engage the enemies that want to crush our spirits, keep us from being wholly integrated and irreparably de-humanize us. Whether it's the abuse we suffered as children, or the abuse we heap upon ourselves with self-destructive behaviors, or even the dysfunctions of our families, businesses and culture—we're in this together. Sharing our successes and failures helps others slay their own dragons."

Everyone was up and moving toward the door. Joshua was staring at Moerae and shaking his head in admiration. "You, woman, are what my mother would have called 'more than a *shenyer punim on a klugger blondeh kop.'*"

Ruth was the only one who laughed. Everyone else looked confused.

"More than a beautiful face on a smart blonde head," he translated.

"More than that, Joshua," Jane said, already laughing. "I'm sure you've been wondering: She is naturally blonde!"

Joshua gasped. Everyone else had known this all along. He roared with laughter from deep in his belly.

"Like I've always said, I'm the last one to know what goes on in this organization. Including who's sleeping with whom."

The best part was it didn't matter.

The war was over.

Epilogue

Like the TV screen staring back at them, Ruth and Joshua sat in muted silence. Had they been able to read the announcer's lips, they would have been aware that a crucial play had just taken place. "Baseball," the announcer was shouting, "is a game of inches!" In excruciating detail and slow motion, the ball's trajectory was being replayed. As the blurry white projectile approached the thin white chalk of the foul line, the high-tech wizardry of television gave millions of couch potatoes a view no normal eye could have ever captured.

The camera lens zoomed in and slowed down the rotating blur even further. A white puff could clearly be seen. The speeding bullet had nicked the foul line. The umpire, a mere mortal surrounded by high technology, had been vindicated. This time he'd made a correct judgment call. The team on the field had suffered a petit mort, the team at bat a moment of joy. A few inches out, and their roles would have been reversed. The umpire's call, "Play ball!" moved the drama on to the next play waiting to unfold—so much like life itself.

Pictures from the last twenty-four hours ran silently through both their minds painfully reminding them that life was also a game of inches. Foul play had cost Damien and Paul their lives. A thermo strip no more than a few inches in length and the eagle eyes of a dedicated colleague had saved both Joshua and his patient.

Whether Joshua's and therefore C.C.A.'s precipitous slide had been arrested in the nick of time remained to be seen. Twenty-twenty hindsight would also be the final judge of whether Peter's knife had cut away the correct few inches of Ruth's breast.

Joshua saw Ruth wince and twist her upper body. "Are you in pain, sweetheart?"

Ruth tucked her chin into her upper chest. She struggled to peer into the small opening where her nightgown was tied together. "No, not really. I'm just afraid about how much Peter had to chop away. Can you tell?" she asked hesitantly. Joshua's hands reached out to untie the top of her gown.

Fingers that had knotted thousands of feet of sutures suddenly felt stiff when confronted by two six-inch strands of silken thread. Joshua was uncertain how much more stark reality his system could stand today. The bow finally came apart.

"He's got it all packed and bandaged, Hon. It's hard to tell."

A tear began to roll down Ruth's cheek. "I just hope it doesn't look too ugly. I'm afraid ... I'm really frightened ... that you won't love me anymore."

A host of false but well-intended clichés flashed across Joshua's mind, the kinds of things he'd said hundreds of times to soothe a patient's fears when he felt totally helpless himself. The words rose to Joshua's lips then were swallowed back down. He struggled to choke back his own tears. He leaned over and planted a warm and tender kiss on Ruth's lips.

After looking deeply into her eyes for a moment, he kissed her bandaged breast. He lifted his head and took her unbounded hand into both of his. "I'm the one who has been ugly. And you'd have every right to ... to ... cut me out of your life."

Ruth released her free hand. Awkwardly reaching up, she stroked his head and ran her fingers through his grey hair. As if moving in slow motion, she brought his head back toward her un-bandaged breast, until she could feel the warmth of his lips on it, then to the bandaged side and back again. She lifted his head and kissed his lips.

"I may be in tight with the ex-boss of this place, but the current boss is also my doctor. He told me to get as much rest as I could. So as soon as you satisfy my curiosity that the letter that fell out of your pocket is not from one of your lovers," she said, "I'm going to boot you out so I can get some shut-eye."

Joshua reached to the floor. Opening the envelope, he filled Ruth in on its history. "I wish I could go back and kiss her good-bye again."

Two pieces of paper dropped out onto the bed. On one was a graphic familiar to both of them. Joshua held it up for Ruth to see. She nodded.

The amazing figure was the one that contains images of both a very young woman and a very old woman—depending on how you look at it. Ruth had pointed out to him the first time she had shown it to Joshua that most people see one or the other. A few gleefully report seeing both images.

"What amazes me," Joshua recalled Ruth saying, "is how hardly anyone reports seeing a person who happens to be female, young or old. Why do we insist on categorizing people by gender age or other characteristics?"

The second piece of paper was the poem Mrs. Wong had promised Joshua her husband would send—the 'tip' she wanted to give him. Joshua leaned back up against Ruth's pillow so she could read it along with him, in mute silence.

What Do You See, Nurses?

What do you see, nurses, what do you see?
What are you thinking when you look at me?
A crabbed old woman, wrinkled and not very wise.
Who dribbles her food and makes no replies?
Who seems not to notice or hear what you say.
And forever loses something every day.

Is that what you're thinking, is that what you see?
Then open your eyes, you're not looking at me.
I'll tell you who I am as I sit here so still,
As I use at your bidding and eat at your will,
I'm a bride at twenty—my heart gives a leap,
Remembering the vows that I promised to keep:
At twenty-five now I have young of my own
Who need me to build a secure happy home;
A woman of thirty my young now grow fast,
Bound to each other with ties that should last;
At forty my young sons have grown and are gone,
But my man's beside me to see I don't mourn;
At fifty, once more babies play round my knee,
Again we know children, my loved one and me;
Dark days are upon me, my husband could soon be dead,
I look at the future and shudder with dread,
I'm an old woman now and nature is cruel-
'Tis her jest to make old age look like a fool.
The body it crumbles, grace and vigor depart,
There is now a stone where I once had a heart.
But inside this old carcass a young girl still dwells,
And now and again my battered heart swells.
I remember the joys, I remember the pain,
And I'm loving and living life over again.
I think of the years all too few—gone too fast,
And accept the stark fact that nothing can last.
So open your eyes, open and see,
Open your heart, look closer—see *me*.